Tickled Pink: A Lighthearted Journey Through the History of Sex Toys

Ava Incite

DWN

DWN Create

Contents

Introduction

Ah, dear reader! You have ventured into the lascivious realm of "Tickled Pink," a titillating tale tracing the tantalizing trajectory of trinkets designed to tickle our most private predilections. These prurient playthings, known as sex toys, have enjoyed a long and illustrious history – one that transcends time and culture – from the frisky forays of our ancient ancestors to the technologically titivated trysts of today.

But before we embark on this rambunctious romp through history, let us first address the blushing elephant in the boudoir: why, you may ask, is such an exploration necessary? To which I say: why not? For too long has this subject been ensconced in hushed whispers and surreptitious giggles. Sex toys are a part of human experience as valid as any other; they deserve their moment in the sun (though perhaps not quite so literally – certain materials are rather sensitive to sunlight, after all).

It is high time we brought these delightful devices out from under the bed and into intellectual discourse. Whether you wield them with wanton abandon or blushingly disavow any knowledge thereof, there is no denying their considerable impact on human sexuality throughout history. So come with me (pun very much intended), and together we shall demystify these prurient playthings.

Now then! Picture yourself at a genteel gathering of acquaintances when suddenly someone cracks wise about "marital aids" or "personal massagers." Titters echo around the room like mischievous sprites; cheeks flush crimson; monocles drop into teacups. This scene illustrates our society's peculiar relationship with sex toys: simultaneously curious yet embarrassed by them.

Our journey begins with an entertaining anecdote involving an unwitting chap who once found himself at such a soirée. Poor Percival Percussive-Penchant was the unfortunate soul who, while searching for a lost cufflink, stumbled upon the hostess's hidden cache of dildos. The mortified matriarch insisted they were part of her "art collection," but the cat was out of the bag (and into the bedroom!). The poor woman was so embarrassed that hid away for the rest of the duration of her own party!

This amusing tale serves as a reminder that we, as a society, must strive to destigmatize conversations about sex toys. After all, if we can openly discuss our predilections for art or music or fine wine (or even cheese), why not our proclivities in private pleasure?

With this in mind, allow me to divulge the aims and aspirations of this most titillating tome: first and foremost, to inform you, dear reader! For what is knowledge but power – and what greater power than that which begets pleasure? Through these pages shall we uncover untold stories of human ingenuity; fascinating facts from bygone eras; titanic tales of triumph and tribulation in pursuit of satisfaction.

Finally – enlightenment! It is our hope that through these chronicles you might gain newfound appreciation for the history embedding these bawdy baubles within broader sexual context. With candid discussions about sexuality woven throughout each chapter like sultry threads binding together tapestries of time; we aspire not only to educate but also inspire self-discovery.

And so begins our journey into the annals (ahem) of sex toy history: from their ancient beginnings in cultures spanning continents, to the impact of religion in medieval times, and the inventive spirit that brought forth rubber and early vibrators. We shall explore the heady days of the sexual revolution, technological advancements in design and materials, and peer into a future where artificial intelligence co-mingles with our most intimate desires.

It is my dearest wish that you emerge from this titillating tour with a newfound respect for these humble instruments of pleasure – their history as rich and varied as the myriad sensations they bring forth.

But enough preamble! It is time to dive headlong into this salacious saga. I extend to you an invitation – nay, a challenge! – to embrace the past, present, and future of sex toys with open arms (and perhaps open legs). Let us embark upon this journey together, armed with curiosity and an unquenchable thirst for knowledge. And above all else: may we find ourselves tickled pink along the way.

Chapter 1: Ancient Beginnings

In the misty and mysterious annals of human history, the pursuit of pleasure has been a perennial preoccupation. Indeed, our ancestors—bless their loins—have bequeathed us a legacy of love-toys that bears witness to their carnal creativity. In this chapter, dear reader, we shall embark upon an odyssey into antiquity in search of the progenitors to our modern playthings.

Our tale commences in the Stone Age—an era that witnessed the birth of mankind's ingenuity in crafting tools for survival, sustenance, and satisfaction. Anthropological excavations have revealed that even amidst a milieu characterized by rawness and brutality, our forebears did not shy away from indulging in sensual delights. Enter stage left: dildos carved from bone and stone.

These rudimentary relics stand as testaments to humanity's eternal quest for pleasure—a veritable Pandora's box (sans calamities) with which we can probe into the sexual psyche of yore. These objects may seem primitive compared to today's silicone symphony; however, they bear witness to our primal yearning for intimacy.

It is said that Neanderthals themselves were quite adept at crafting these early playthings—for who better understood their needs than those who experienced them firsthand? Eve surely felt Adam wasn't enough! Even Cleopatra was rumored to have partaken in Copulation Machinations (as they were once known) by filling hollow gourds with bees whose buzzing would induce sensations akin to divine vibrations.

The purpose and significance of these Stone Age dildos are manifold; foremost among them is their contribution to procreation rituals wherein virility was celebrated with gusto. It is believed that these devices were employed by women who wished to conceive but lacked male consorts at hand—an ingenious solution conjured up by necessity and desire.

But let us not forget that humans have forever been social creatures; hence it would be remiss if we overlooked the communal aspect inherent within these early sex toys. Dildos also functioned as talismans against evil spirits and maladies—a role akin to those fulfilled by fertility figurines whose voluptuous forms served as vessels for divine intervention.

As regards materials used in crafting these titillating trinkets, one cannot help but marvel at the artisanal mastery displayed by our ancestors. Bones, stones, and even antlers were meticulously sculpted into pleasing shapes—evidence of a creative flair that straddled the line between utility and artistry.

These Stone Age sculptors, no doubt fueled by their own passion for pleasure-seeking pursuits, harnessed the inherent qualities of their chosen materials to fashion objects that could both withstand vigorous use and tantalize the senses. The hardness of stone imbued these early dildos with an unyielding quality that must have resonated with users who craved intensity in their intimate encounters.

Now we must shift our gaze from the rugged landscapes of prehistory to the sun-kissed shores of Ancient Greece—a realm teeming with gods and demigods who reveled in carnal delights. It is within this milieu that we encounter olisbos—devices fashioned from leather, wood, or stone—that would come to be known as "dildos."

The cultural and social context of olisbos in Ancient Greece cannot be overstated; after all, this was an age when sensuality was celebrated rather than shunned. Both men and women partook in pleasure-seeking activities as a means to connect with one another (and themselves) on a deeper level.

In fact, it was not uncommon for Athenian women to gather at parties wherein they would unabashedly discuss matters pertaining to sex—including their fondness for these phallic playthings. As such gatherings often culminated in playful exchanges of olisbos among attendees; one can imagine them engaged in spirited debates regarding size preferences or trading tips on techniques for optimal enjoyment.

Of course, there exists another dimension to olisbos—one steeped in religious symbolism and ritualistic practices. To comprehend this aspect fully requires immersing ourselves within the mythological tapestry woven throughout Ancient Greek civilization.

A tale that comes to mind is of Lysistrata, the play by Aristophanes, wherein women wield their olisbos as a form of rebellion—refusing to indulge in carnal relations with their husbands until peace was restored between warring city-states. Oh, how history repeats itself when men are left wanting!

Indeed, many scholars posit that olisbos played a crucial role in the worship of Dionysus—the god of ecstasy and intoxication. As partakers in his cult indulged in unbridled revelry, it is believed that these phallic symbols were employed as conduits for channeling divine energy.

Moreover, olisbos also figured prominently within the Eleusinian Mysteries—a series of secret rites reserved for initiates who sought communion with the goddess Demeter. During these enigmatic ceremonies, participants wielded olisbos to invoke her fertility powers—thus ensuring a bountiful harvest.

In summation, our journey into antiquity has unveiled a world wherein sex toys were revered as both pleasure-inducing implements and sacred instruments capable of transcending mundane reality. From the Stone Age to Ancient Greece, humanity's penchant for erotic exploration remains a constant theme—one that shall resonate throughout subsequent chapters as we delve further into this titillating topic.

Thus concludes our initial foray into the annals of sex toy history; yet rest assured dear reader, there exists a veritable treasure trove awaiting us just beyond the horizon—a trove overflowing with tales of passion and playthings from ages past. So gird your loins and prepare to be tickled pink as we embark upon an odyssey unlike any other!

Chapter 2: The Jade Age of China

Allow me to whisk you away to the land of dragons and emperors, where ancient wisdom coalesced with human ingenuity to create objects of pleasure that have stood the test of time. Yes, we are venturing into the mystical realm of Ancient China, an empire whose contributions to the world extend far beyond its Great Wall.

As we delve into this chapter about jade pleasure plugs and early Ben Wa balls, let me first regale you with a tale that illustrates how Chinese culture has been a veritable treasure trove for historians and pleasure seekers alike. Once upon a time in an illustrious dynasty long ago—or perhaps not so long ago when one considers the grand scheme of history—a Chinese emperor was said to have had at his disposal a cabinet filled with an assortment of jade sex toys intended for use by himself and his many concubines. Legend has it that these delicate instruments were so expertly crafted that they could elicit cries of ecstasy from even the most stoic courtesan.

Now that your appetite is suitably whetted, let us explore further the significance of jade in Ancient Chinese culture and its connection to their erotic artifacts.

In ancient China, few materials were held in higher esteem than jade. This precious gemstone was often associated with purity and moral integrity, making it more valuable than gold or silver in certain circles. So esteemed was jade in fact that it became ingrained within Chinese mythology itself: It is said that Xi Wangmu (the Queen Mother of the West) resided in her Jade Palace atop Kunlun Mountain—a location signifying both spiritual transcendence and earthly delight.

But fear not! Our purpose here is not merely an exposition on geology or mythology but rather on how this wondrous material came to be used for titillation as well as piety. The ancient Chinese believed that jade contained within it a potent life force akin to the human soul or spirit. By fashioning pleasure objects from this divine material, they sought to imbue their intimate encounters with an aura of sacredness and spiritual energy.

One can only imagine the delight experienced by ancient Chinese lovers as they gazed upon their jade pleasure plugs, glinting in the moonlight like tiny celestial bodies. These meticulously carved tokens of affection would then be gently introduced into their most secret of chambers, where they would serve not only as instruments of pleasure but also as conduits for that ineffable life force known as qi (pronounced "chee"). Thus, in one fell swoop—a phrase I use here with utmost care—the ancients transformed their carnal passions into a transcendent communion with the divine.

With such heavenly connotations in mind, it is no wonder that these jade artifacts have captured our collective imagination for millennia. But let us now shift our focus from these celestial playthings to another invention from this fertile period: the enigmatic Ben Wa balls.

Before we delve into the function and purpose of Ben Wa balls in Ancient Chinese society, allow me to clarify any confusion surrounding these beguiling spheres. You may be familiar with them under various aliases—geisha balls or love beads among others—but rest assured that all refer to those same small orbs designed for insertion into one's most intimate regions.

The origins of Ben Wa balls are shrouded in mystery, much like the veils worn by many a concubine who might have employed them during her amorous encounters. Though some historians attribute their invention to Japanese geishas (thus adding yet another layer of intrigue), there is ample evidence suggesting that they were first utilized by women in Ancient China.

In those days when women were often relegated to more subservient roles, Ben Wa balls served as a means for them to assert control over their own sexual pleasure. By inserting these spheres—often made of jade or other precious materials—into their nether regions, women were able to discreetly engage in an erotic dance with themselves, wherein the gentle motions of the balls would provide a most delightful internal caress.

Yet there was more to Ben Wa balls than just pure pleasure seeking. In Ancient China, it was believed that a woman's sexual energy played a crucial role in her overall health and vitality. These small orbs were thought to harness and cultivate this energy, thus promoting not only sensual satisfaction but also physical well-being.

But let us not forget the role that men played in this lascivious tale! For you see, the use of Ben Wa balls was not confined solely to the boudoirs of Chinese courtesans. Indeed, many an amorous gentleman found delight in employing these tantalizing toys during his trysts, often inserting them into his partner before engaging in other activities—a veritable game of hide-and-seek where both participants stood to win.

In this way then did Ben Wa balls become an indispensable tool for lovers throughout Ancient China—a symbol not only of sensual pleasure but also spiritual connection and mutual satisfaction between partners.

As we conclude our exploration of Ancient China's jade pleasure plugs and early Ben Wa balls, I trust that you have been titillated by these tales from yesteryear. May they serve as a testament to human ingenuity and our ceaseless quest for pleasure—an endeavor that transcends time and place. And remember: When next you gaze upon a piece of jade or feel the weighty heft of those beguiling spheres within your palm—I speak here metaphorically; one must exercise proper restraint when discussing such delicate matters—consider their storied past and pay homage to those who came before us on this most delightful journey of discovery.

Chapter 3: Ancient Impact of Sex Toys

In our arousing odyssey through the annals of pleasure, we now find ourselves delving into the social and cultural significance of sex toys in ancient civilizations. Oh, what a titillating tale it is! For, dear reader, you shall soon discover that our ancestors were not merely preoccupied with their humble survival; they also devoted considerable time and energy to the pursuit of bodily delights. From religion to medicine, gender dynamics to power plays – all facets of ancient society bore witness to the influence of these marvelous instruments.

Firstly, let us examine the role sex toys played in religious and spiritual practices. It may seem rather peculiar that objects designed for carnal gratification should have any association with matters divine; yet history reveals that many cultures incorporated such items into their rituals and worship.

In ancient Egypt – a civilization renowned for its sexual openness – phallic objects were held in high regard as symbols of fertility and life-giving potency. Priests would anoint stone dildos with sacred oils before placing them upon altars as offerings to deities such as Min (the god of procreation) or Hathor (the goddess of love). These blessed trinkets then became imbued with mystical properties, believed to bestow blessings upon those who sought their intimate embrace.

Ancient India was similarly enamored with sex toys' spiritual potential. According to Hindu tradition, lingams (stylized phalluses) symbolize Lord Shiva's generative prowess; they remain an object of veneration today within temples across the subcontinent. Tantric practitioners also employed various devices during their esoteric love-making sessions – achieving union with one's partner whilst utilizing a sacred instrument was thought to bring about transcendental bliss.

The use of sex toys extended beyond mere symbolism or ritualistic enhancement; indeed, many ancient societies believed that these items possessed genuine curative powers. For instance, the Greeks and Romans were known to employ olisbos (or dildos) in the treatment of a malady referred to as "hysteria." This mysterious ailment – primarily afflicting women, naturally – was characterized by an assortment of vague symptoms, including anxiety, irritability, and sexual frustration.

The ancient physician Galen postulated that hysteria resulted from a "wandering womb," which could only be coaxed back into its proper position through vigorous stimulation. Thus, doctors would prescribe olisbos – often crafted from smooth materials such as glass or polished wood – for their patients' self-administered therapy. And while modern medical science has since debunked this peculiar hypothesis regarding uterine vagrancy, we must nevertheless applaud our forebears' ingenuity in devising creative solutions to life's carnal challenges.

Another fascinating aspect of sex toys' role in ancient societies is their impact on gender dynamics and power relations. It is no secret that throughout history, women have often found themselves at the mercy of patriarchal norms; their sexual pleasure frequently dismissed or marginalized in favor of male satisfaction. Yet these cunning contrivances offered our ancestresses an opportunity to seize control over their own erotic destinies.

Similarly empowering were strap-on devices utilized by certain Greek women during Dionysian revelries. These bacchanalian celebrations revolved around ecstatic dancing and copious consumption of wine; they also featured scenes of uninhibited eroticism wherein traditional gender roles were gleefully subverted. Women donning leather phalluses would engage in mock sexual encounters with men or other women, thereby reveling in the temporary reversal of power that these artificial appendages bestowed upon them.

Yet it must be noted that the use of sex toys was not always a liberating force for women throughout ancient times. In some instances, they served to uphold and reinforce existing hierarchies. For example, Chinese noblemen were known to employ jade pleasure plugs – inserted into their wives' vaginas – as a means of asserting ownership and control over their bodies; the ornate carvings adorning these items signified status and wealth, while also functioning as an erotic chastity belt.

Furthermore, phallic objects have frequently been employed as symbols of male dominance across various cultures. The Romans revered the god Priapus, whose gigantic member was said to bring abundance and prosperity; statues bearing his likeness would be placed within gardens or at crossroads to ward off evil spirits (and perhaps make passersby feel rather inadequate). Such displays can be understood as visual reminders of patriarchal authority – a message that continues to reverberate through modern sculpture and art.

In conclusion, our examination of sex toys' social and cultural significance reveals a rich tapestry woven from threads both empowering and oppressive. These delightful devices have enabled individuals throughout history to explore new realms of sensuality while simultaneously challenging societal norms. And yet they also serve as reminders that sexuality is often shackled by convention – particularly when it comes to gender roles and power dynamics.

As we continue our journey through time, let us bear in mind this complex legacy: for every tale of liberation wrought by these marvelous contraptions, there remains another wherein such objects are wielded as instruments of control. In doing so, we can better appreciate not only how far we've come but also how much work remains in dismantling antiquated attitudes towards pleasure-seeking pursuits.

Thus ends our sojourn into antiquity; now let us venture forth into the murky waters of the Middle Ages, where we shall witness the interplay between religion and eroticism – an unlikely coupling that yields most intriguing results. So, strap yourselves in (or on, as it were), dear readers; our lascivious locomotive rumbles ever onwards!

Chapter 4: The Middle Ages and Renaissance

As we saunter through the annals of history, it is nigh impossible to overlook the significant role played by religion in shaping societies' attitudes towards the pleasures of the flesh. The Middle Ages and Renaissance were periods marked by a profound influence of religion on every aspect of life, including sexual matters. It was during these ages that Christianity rose to prominence, casting its divine light upon all things carnal.

The impact of Christianity on attitudes towards sex toys cannot be overstated. Forsooth, this sacred institution considered such pleasure-inducing contraptions as abominations against nature itself. With their strict moral code and zealous pursuit for purity, Christian leaders were keen to put a damper on any activities that might lead their flock astray from righteousness.

The medieval Church viewed sexuality as a necessary evil – an unfortunate consequence of humanity's fall from grace in the Garden of Eden. Intercourse was deemed acceptable solely for procreation purposes within holy matrimony; any other form of erotic dalliance was frowned upon as sinful indulgence. Thus, sex toys found themselves banished to the shadows as taboo implements designed purely for lascivious gratification.

It must be mentioned here that not all forms of Christianity adopted the same stance on matters pertaining to intimacy. In fact, some denominations even embraced sexual expression in more libertine ways than one might expect given their overarching devotion to piety.

Nevertheless, 'tis undeniable that Christian dogma played an instrumental role in stigmatizing and marginalizing sex toy use throughout much of Europe during these eras. This opprobrium extended not only to those who wielded such devices but also to artisans who crafted these tools de amour – many faced persecution or excommunication if discovered partaking in this ignoble profession.

In addition to disseminating stigma surrounding sex toys via religious teachings, the Church also sought to regulate their use more directly by wielding its considerable influence over secular powers. The ecclesiastical establishment often collaborated with monarchs and other political authorities to enforce strict measures against the sale, possession, or utilization of these pleasure-providing contraptions.

Take for example, the infamous case of one hapless merchant in fifteenth-century France who found himself caught amidst a whirlwind of controversy for attempting to peddle his illicit wares. This purveyor of carnal delights was apprehended by zealous clergymen and subsequently dragged before a tribunal, where he faced charges of heresy and immorality – all because he dared to hawk "demonically inspired" sex toys made from leather and wood.

In another instance, an enterprising Italian craftsman narrowly escaped excommunication after being accused of producing "devilish instruments" designed solely for self-pleasure. Fortunately for this artisan (and his customers), some influential clerics intervened on his behalf, arguing that such devices could serve medicinal purposes if used under appropriate guidance.

It is worth noting that despite these ardent efforts to quash the spread of sex toys during the Middle Ages and Renaissance periods, they continued to exist – albeit furtively – within society's seamy underbelly. The resilient human spirit yearned for pleasure even in the face of moral condemnation; henceforth individuals clandestinely procured these objects d'amour via secretive transactions or crafted them surreptitiously at home using rudimentary materials.

As we meander through this epoch filled with religious fervor mingled with artistic expression, it is crucial not only to consider how Christianity influenced attitudes towards sex toys but also how art itself reflected society's perceptions regarding these objects. Indeed, both literature and visual arts during this time period frequently depicted scenes involving amorous encounters between lovers – occasionally featuring erotic accessories that would be deemed scandalous by today's standards.

It is in the hallowed halls of Renaissance art where we find titillating glimpses into the clandestine world of carnal pleasure. Works such as "The Garden of Earthly Delights" by Hieronymus Bosch and "Venus and Cupid" by Lorenzo Lotto showcase a fascinating mix of sensuality, passion, and hidden elements that hint at the existence of sex toys during this era.

In written form, too, we find evidence aplenty that such implements were not entirely absent from society's consciousness. The infamous libertine Pietro Aretino penned a series of irreverent sonnets that dared to extol the joys brought forth by dildos – an act for which he faced both admiration and censure from his contemporaries.

Thus, while Christianity might have endeavored to cast an austere pall over matters related to sexuality (and sex toys in particular), it could not entirely suppress humanity's innate desire for self-expression and sensual gratification. This tension between religious dogma and corporeal appetite would continue to play out through subsequent historical epochs – laying the groundwork for the complex relationship between sex toys and society that persists even today.

One must marvel at how our forebears covertly pursued their desires amidst such repressive conditions — perhaps taking inspiration from those who dared risk excommunication or worse simply so they might satisfy their carnal curiosities with delightful devices fashioned from wood or leather. For verily it is said: Where there is will, there's a way (or in this case, a dildo).

The Middle Ages may have seen fit to consign these playthings to furtive shadows; however, fear not! As history marched on - much like those ingenious medieval lovers - mankind would continue finding novel means with which to indulge its innate yearning for sensual pleasure. Thus did sex toys persevere against all odds: Stashed away in secret compartments or cunningly crafted using primitive materials, these trusty tools of titillation awaited the time when libertine sensibilities might once more flourish unfettered by the fetters of piety and hypocrisy.

As we shall see in subsequent chapters, our tale of sex toys is replete with heroes and villains: From bawdy poets who penned paeans to pleasure-giving implements to puritanical zealots intent on eradicating carnal "corruption" from their midst. And through it all, ever resilient, the humble sex toy persisted — an unflagging beacon of sensual satisfaction amidst a sea of religious sanctimony and repression.

Let us then raise our goblets to toast those intrepid souls whose courageous pursuit for carnal pleasure helped ensure that future generations might enjoy the fruits (and dildos) of their labor. For as history teaches us, even in the face of adversity one can always find solace between sheets... or within secret drawers where naughty contraptions lay hidden from prying eyes.

So let us revel in humanity's colorful past as we trace the thread (or perhaps more accurately, vibrator cord) that has led us from medieval times to our modern world - a world teeming with delightfully sinful inventions designed for nothing less than pure blissful ecstasy. And mayhap some day soon readers will look back upon our age with equal fascination – wondering how such ingeniously lewd gadgets were ever considered taboo at all!

Chapter 5: The Hollow Phallus

As we gallivant through the annals of history, it is incumbent upon us to stop for a moment and examine the Middle Ages and Renaissance - that pivotal epoch when mankind's exploration of carnal pleasure found itself in a delightful dance with medical progress. So come hither and let us delve into the invention of that most curious contraption: the "hollow phallus." To elucidate this peculiar phenomenon, we shall peruse its development as a medical tool and uncover how it ensconced itself within the praxis of physicians during those turbulent times.

As you may recall from our previous disquisitions, sex toys have been no stranger to human civilization throughout its storied past. The hollow phallus emerged from this rich tradition as an innovative response to certain biological conundrums faced by men and women alike in their quest for procreation or merely pleasure-seeking adventures. Allow me to expound further.

The development of the hollow phallus owes much to those intrepid medieval doctors who sought new ways not only to treat but also understand ailments plaguing their patients' nether regions. In particular, these avant-garde healers discovered that some women suffered from what was then known as "hysteria" – a vexing condition whose symptoms included nervousness, irritability, insomnia and (gasp!) even sexual desire on occasion. And so it was that these astute clinicians deduced that stimulation of the afflicted woman's genitalia might offer respite from her suffering.

Armed with this insight into feminine maladies - which would surely make Sigmund Freud himself blush like a schoolchild at her first ball - enterprising physicians crafted artificial penises fashioned out of various materials such as leather or glass. These devices were then filled with warm water or other concoctions designed to simulate ejaculation when strategically deployed within a woman's vagina. Medical practitioners believed that the introduction of this faux seminal fluid would help to alleviate symptoms associated with hysteria by inducing a state of blissful relaxation, known as "paroxysm."

The hollow phallus was not confined to the treatment of hysteria alone. Indeed, it also came to be employed as an aid for men suffering from erectile dysfunction or other maladies that prevented them from performing their conjugal duties. In some instances, these ingenious contraptions were used as surrogates when a husband was away on military campaigns or pilgrimage, ensuring that his wife's needs were addressed in absentia.

As the Renaissance dawned and humankind emerged from the long winter of medieval darkness with renewed vigor - their minds ablaze with inquisitiveness and creativity - so too did our beloved hollow phallus evolve. Those innovative souls who dared to dream beyond the confines of contemporary wisdom forged ever more elaborate versions of these devices out of metals such as bronze or silver, even going as far as to adorn them with precious stones or intricate carvings. Such ostentatious accouterments surely made those stiff members feel like veritable kings amongst their organ brethren!

Now you may wonder how prevalent these hollow phalli were in medical practices during this period – and rightly so! For what better way is there to gauge the impact something has had upon history than by measuring its ubiquity? And thus, I shall regale you with tales and tidbits about these fascinating objects and their place within the annals of medicine.

In truth, it is difficult for us modern-day pleasure enthusiasts (and historians) to ascertain precisely how widespread the use of hollow phalli was in medical practice during the Middle Ages and Renaissance. However, we can surmise that they occupied a prominent role based on evidence gleaned from various sources - including art, literature, and surviving artifacts themselves.

For instance, several illuminated manuscripts from this era depict physicians administering the hollow phallus to female patients, suggesting that this treatment was held in high regard by medical professionals of the time. In some cases, these images reveal a surprising level of detail about how these devices were manufactured and deployed - no doubt providing many a medieval doctor with an invaluable visual reference guide.

Literature of the period also provides us with tantalizing clues about the prevalence of hollow phalli in medical practice. Prominent writers such as Giovanni Boccaccio (of "The Decameron" fame) and Geoffrey Chaucer (author of "The Canterbury Tales") make mention of such devices within their works - thereby immortalizing them for posterity and ensuring that countless generations would be privy to their existence.

Moreover, archaeological excavations have unearthed numerous examples of hollow phalli from sites across Europe, lending further credence to our belief that they were indeed widely employed by practitioners during this epoch. Some well-preserved specimens can even be found on display in museums today - offering visitors an intimate glimpse into the world of medieval and Renaissance medicine.

It is clear then that the hollow phallus was not merely a frivolous plaything or passing fancy but rather occupied a significant place within the annals of medical history during those tumultuous times. As we continue our journey through mankind's storied exploration of sexual pleasure, let us pause for a moment to appreciate how far we have come since those days when brave men and women dared to dream beyond convention in pursuit of health and happiness.

And so it is with bated breath that I invite you to accompany me further down this titillating path as we uncover more secrets about our ancestors' most intimate desires – all in the name of enlightenment and understanding, of course. For as we peer into the looking glass of history, we shall find that our forebears were not so dissimilar from ourselves in their quest for pleasure – a reassuring revelation that serves to remind us of all that, indeed, the human spirit remains ever constant.

Thus concludes our exploration into the fascinating world of hollow phallus during the Middle Ages and Renaissance. Through art, literature, archaeological finds, and anecdotes aplenty, we have seen how these ingenious contraptions became an indispensable tool for medical practitioners seeking to alleviate various ailments related to sexual health. As we venture forth into subsequent chapters chronicling mankind's pursuit of satisfaction through sex toys across time and space, let us bear in mind this crucial episode in our collective past - a testament to human ingenuity and perseverance in the face of adversity.

For even as plague ravaged populations and wars rent continents asunder during those dark days (and nights), humans never lost sight of their capacity for pleasure or their innate desire to seek solace through physical intimacy - be it with partners or artificial aids. And thus, it is with renewed ardor that I bid you farewell until next time when once more we shall delve deep into history's boudoir – eager voyeurs privy to pleasures long past yet eternally relevant.

Chapter 6: Early Portrayal of Sex Toys

The Middle Ages and Renaissance period, a time of fervent artistry and intellectual pursuits, also bore witness to an undercurrent of sensual expression that manifested itself in erotic art and literature. This chapter shall endeavor to explore the portrayal of sex toys in the creative realms during this era, examining their impact on popularity and acceptance amidst a society bound by religious stringency.

Within the shadows of grand cathedrals and ornate castles that graced Europe during these times, artists dared to challenge conventions with their paintbrushes or quills. They breathed life into lascivious images that drew inspiration from ancient texts such as Ovid's "Ars Amatoria" (The Art of Love) or tales from Boccaccio's "Decameron." These works not only titillated readers with their amorous exploits but also showcased various implements employed for plea-sure-seeking adventures.

As one delves deeper into this intriguing world, it becomes apparent that sex toys were not merely figments conjured up by modern-day manufacturers; rather they enjoyed a rich history woven intricately within the fabric of human development. To truly appreciate these salacious gems hidden amidst great cultural achievements, we must first journey through the artistic landscape where they made their mark.

The portrayal of sex toys in Renaissance-era artwork serves as ev-idence that objects designed for carnal delights held undeniable in-trigue for those who dared depict them. One such artist was Giulio Romano, known for his masterful frescoes adorning Villa Lante al Gianicolo – a testament to hedonistic fulfillment. Amongst scenes teeming with voluptuous nymphs and satyrs engaged in amorous pur-suits were images featuring dildos crafted from materials ranging from wood to glass.

Another notable example is Agostino Carracci's series entitled "Lascivie," where the artist depicted various couples in intimate acts, showcasing an assortment of pleasure devices. Indeed, his works bear witness to the wide array of sex toys permeating the era – a testimony that they were not only used but also incorporated into artistic ex-pression.

The literary realm did not shy away from exploring these sensu-al topics either. In fact, some of the most celebrated authors found inspiration in erotic themes and imagery, weaving tales filled with seduction and desire while also shedding light on the role sex toys played during this period. François Rabelais' "Gargantua and Panta-gruel," for instance, featured a memorable passage wherein Panurge presents a collection of dildos crafted from diverse materials to delight his companion's carnal senses.

Another example is John Cleland's notorious novel "Fanny Hill," which recounts the amorous escapades of its eponymous heroine as she encounters various sexual aids throughout her journey (albeit set in later 18th-century England). These depictions underscored society's fascination with erotic pleasures and served to raise awareness about sex toys as objects designed for mutual gratification.

It is crucial to acknowledge that despite their prevalence within artistic circles, these depictions often faced resistance from religious authorities who sought to suppress expressions deemed immoral or obscene. Nevertheless, artists and writers continued their subversive endeavors by cloaking them within allegory or symbolism – an attempt at circumventing censorship while simultaneously indulging their own desires for creative freedom.

Considering this context, one can surmise that erotic art indeed played a significant role in shaping public perception towards sex toys during this era. By incorporating them into visual narratives or poetic verses brimming with sensuality and passion, these creatives succeeded in challenging societal norms while also expanding upon human understanding of pleasure-seeking pursuits.

The impact of erotic art on sex toy popularity and acceptance during the Renaissance cannot be overstated. For many individuals living under ecclesiastical rule, these works served as a clandestine window into a world of carnal delights – one that dared to celebrate the human form and its boundless capacity for pleasure.

This newfound awareness inevitably paved the way for greater acceptance of sex toys within certain circles. Despite facing resistance from religious authorities or conservative factions, those who embraced erotic art also developed an appreciation for the objects featured therein – recognizing their potential to enhance intimacy and heighten sensation.

As a result, one could argue that this era laid the foundations for contemporary attitudes towards sex toys: viewing them not as shameful or perverse, but rather as instruments designed to bring joy and fulfillment within consensual relationships. By appreciating their historical significance and acknowledging their presence amidst some of humanity's greatest artistic achievements, we can begin to dismantle lingering stigmas surrounding these objects while embracing their role in our ongoing quest for pleasure.

The Middle Ages and Renaissance period proved to be a pivotal time in shaping societal perceptions towards sex toys through erotic art and literature. The daring expressions that emerged during this era not only challenged prevailing norms but also contributed significantly to our understanding of human desire.

By delving into the annals of history, we can better appreciate how far society has come in destigmatizing sex toys – acknowledging their role in promoting sexual health and happiness while celebrating their rich heritage. As we journey forward into new realms of technological innovation or bold artistic expressionism, let us remember those who came before us – pioneering creatives who dared to explore uncharted territories with unabashed gusto. It is through this lens that we can truly appreciate our titillating past while embracing an equally tantalizing future filled with pleasure-seeking pursuits.

Chapter 7: Erotic Novels

The pages of history are replete with instances of human innovation, and while the Industrial Revolution spawned a myriad of magnificent machines, it also gave rise to an underappreciated, yet equally consequential invention – the modern sex toy. Indeed, it is during the 18th and 19th centuries that our collective libido experienced a veritable reawakening as our ancestors delved ever deeper into their carnal desires. The burgeoning world of erotic literature played a crucial role in fueling this sensual exploration, leaving no stone – or orifice – unturned in its quest to titillate readers and forever change the way society viewed pleasure products.

As we saunter through this sordid era's boudoirs, let us first examine the circumstances surrounding the emergence of erotic literature. Ah yes, dear reader, for within these lascivious tomes lay tales so salacious as to make even Casanova himself blush like a virgin bride on her wedding night.

No account would be complete without mention of one particularly notorious novel: "Fanny Hill or Memoirs of a Woman of Pleasure" by John Cleland (1748). A scandalous narrative chronicling Fanny's ribald exploits as she navigates London's sexual underworld; this tome proved itself both an incendiary work that ignited heated debates about morality whilst simultaneously arousing many a curious reader.

Despite society's prudish façade at that time, clandestine presses churned out these voluptuous volumes like rabbits breeding beneath silken sheets. As such libidinous texts spread throughout Europe faster than mercury in an ill-prepared syringe (a common treatment for venereal diseases during those halcyon days), underground bookshops specializing in erotic texts blossomed like aphrodisiacal flowers. In France, the notorious Marquis de Sade penned his infamous works, such as "The 120 Days of Sodom" (1785), which celebrated debauchery on a scale heretofore unimaginable.

Across the pond, America too experienced a surge in amorous appetite. With titillating tales like "Venus in Boston: A Romance of City Life" (1849) and "The Libertine's Friend; or Advice to Young Ladies," our colonial cousins eagerly embraced the new world of carnality.

It was during this era that erotic literature not only transformed into an art form but also served as a catalyst for sexual exploration and innovation. Readers found themselves thrust headfirst – if you'll pardon the expression – into lascivious worlds where voluptuous vixens and dashing cads indulged their every whim with abandon.

As these bawdy books infiltrated society like a scintillating rash spreading across one's nether regions, they inadvertently fanned the flames of desire for pleasure products hitherto unknown by most respectable folk. Indeed, erotic literature proved itself both stimulant and instruction manual – providing readers not only with lascivious accounts to whet their appetites but also detailed descriptions of devices designed to bring these fantasies to life.

The pages of such literary masterpieces often featured rapturous accounts involving various forms of phallic paraphernalia which left readers panting for more than just ink-stained fingertips. These titillating tales served as inspiration for inventive individuals who sought to craft contrivances capable of replicating such mind-bending ecstasy within their own boudoirs.

Our journey through history takes us first to England where industrious artisans began crafting dildos from materials such as wood, leather, and even ivory for those with more opulent tastes. As knowledge of these pleasure products spread via word of mouth and clandestine advertisements within erotic novels themselves, the appetite for such devices grew insatiable.

Interestingly, it was not just women who sought solace in the comforting embrace of a well-crafted dildo; many men also found themselves drawn to these delightful devices. Indeed, accounts abound of gentlemen procuring hollow phallic apparatuses designed to aid them in satisfying their partners whilst simultaneously sparing their own virile virtue from the ravages of venereal disease.

Meanwhile, over in France, where hedonism has long been elevated to an art form – or at least a national pastime – talented artisans began crafting elegant "godemichets" from materials such as glass and porcelain. French nobility delighted in gifting one another these beautiful pleasure products which were often disguised as innocuous objects d'art so that they might be displayed proudly on mantelpieces without fear of discovery by prying eyes.

As society's appetite for carnal knowledge continued to grow unabated like an untamed stallion rutting through an open field of dewy grass beneath a full moon's lascivious gaze – yes dear reader, I apologize for my tendency towards poetic digression – sex toys began to evolve at an unprecedented pace. Inventions such as Dr. George Taylor's steam-powered "Manipulator" (1869) emerged during this period seeking to address the ever-growing demands for mechanical feats capable of delivering unparalleled satisfaction.

And so it was that amidst this sumptuous banquet of debauchery and decadence prepared by our 18th and 19th-century ancestors that erotic literature emerged not only as salacious dessert but also a veritable instruction manual on how best to navigate this brave new world teeming with sexual delights hitherto unimagined. It is within these pages that we find the origins of our modern-day fascination with pleasure products – proof positive that while the human species may have come a long way from its primitive past, our appetite for sensual gratification remains as voracious as ever.

Chapter 8

Chapter 8: Well Hello Rubber!

As the world embarked upon a period of immense scientific discovery and technological innovation during the 18th and 19th centuries, so too did it witness the creation of new materials that would prove instrumental in shaping the future of sex toys. One such material was rubber, which not only revolutionized numerous industries but also left an indelible mark on the pleasure product industry.

The history and development of rubber as a material begins with its humble origins as latex sap harvested from wild trees in South America. Indigenous peoples utilized this natural substance for centuries to waterproof their clothing, create balls for games, and even craft primitive prophylactics – foreshadowing its more intimate applications.

It was not until the mid-18th century that European explorers chanced upon this remarkable material while traversing through these foreign lands, delightfully dubbing it "caoutchouc," after the indigenous term "caa-o-chu." At the right time, this versatile substance earned its modern moniker – "rubber" – after English chemist Joseph Priestley discovered its ability to rub out pencil marks. Ah, those were simpler times!

Rubber's transformation into a darling of industrial manufacturing can be credited to Thomas Hancock's invention of mastication (not to be confused with masticating one's dinner) in 1820. This process involved softening raw rubber by heating it and then mechanically working it into a more pliable state, allowing for greater ease in shaping and molding.

However, early rubber products were susceptible to extreme temperatures that either hardened or liquefied them - clearly suboptimal characteristics for objects intended to provide sensual pleasure! Enter American inventor Charles Goodyear. No relation to tires (yet), his serendipitous discovery of vulcanization in 1839 involved adding sulfur to rubber, thus creating a far more robust and long-lasting material. And just like that, rubber bounced into the mainstream.

The use of rubber in the creation of sex toys during the 18th and 19th centuries was nothing short of revolutionary. This pliable new material offered an unparalleled alternative to its predecessors - wood, stone, ivory, and glass - affording users increased flexibility (in every sense) and comfort.

As news of rubber's miraculous properties spread through polite society like wildfire (or a more titillating metaphor), enterprising artisans seized upon this opportunity to craft truly bespoke pleasure products for their discerning clientele. These early incarnations of rubber sex toys were often handcrafted with intricate detailing designed to tantalize both visually and physically – think ornate phalluses adorned with baroque flourishes that would make even the most stoic Victorian matron blush.

However, it is worth noting that these early personal massagers were not without their shortcomings; given the limitations in manufacturing techniques at that time, such creations were prone to imperfections or inconsistencies in texture – one might encounter an unexpected bump along the way! Nevertheless, as technology advanced throughout the 19th century so did our ancestors' love affair with all things rubber - including their pleasure products.

Our journey into this fascinating epoch would be incomplete without delving into another remarkable invention: early vibrators and their "medical" applications. In contrast to widespread belief today that vibrators are devices intended solely for self-gratification or partnered delight, they originally took center stage as veritable medical miracles purported to cure various ailments plaguing women at the time.

The invention and development of early vibrators for medical purposes can be traced back to Dr. Joseph Mortimer Granville, a British physician who first introduced his electro-mechanical vibrator in 1880. Initially designed as a treatment for male muscular pain (an unintentional foreshadowing of its potential power, perhaps?), Dr. Granville soon found that his contraption held tremendous promise for alleviating a widespread female malady – hysteria.

Though the term "hysteria" has long been relegated to the annals of medical history, it was once considered a legitimate diagnosis for women who exhibited symptoms ranging from anxiety and irritability to fainting spells and inexplicable sensations in their... ahem, nether regions. In an era, rife with sexual repression and prudish mores, doctors were quick to prescribe "pelvic massage" as the cure du jour for this mysterious ailment. And so began an intimate relationship between physicians and their patients - one might even call it manual labor.

However, these therapeutic endeavors were both time-consuming and physically demanding for our intrepid healers. Enter the vibrator - a marvel of modern ingenuity! With Dr. Granville's invention in hand (and other places), doctors could now administer treatment with unmatched efficiency, relieving their patients' symptoms while reducing their own fatigue. It was truly a win-win situation!

The evolution of vibrators as sexual pleasure products may have begun under the guise of medical necessity; however, as this newfangled device gained popularity among women eager to explore its more carnal applications, society began to take note.

Early vibrators came in various shapes and sizes - some resembling familiar phallic forms while others bore closer resemblance to household appliances or scientific instruments than tools of titillation. These contraptions offered women newfound agency in exploring their sexuality within the confines of societal expectations.

Yet it would be remiss not to mention that such discretion came at a steep price; these mechanical marvels were luxury items available only to those with deep pockets who could afford such clandestine indulgences - think grande dames sipping tea from fine china while discussing the merits of different vibratory frequencies.

As we venture further into the 19th century, we begin to see a shift in attitudes towards these pleasure products. No longer mere medical instruments or symbols of decadence, vibrators and other devices began to shed their stigma as they became increasingly popular among women of all social strata.

The burgeoning feminist movement of the time played a crucial role in this transformation, pushing for greater openness around female sexuality and encouraging women to take control of their own bodies. Slowly but surely, society began to accept – even embrace – the notion that women were entitled to experience sexual pleasure on their own terms.

And so, concludes our titillating tour through the 18th and 19th centuries - an era marked by invention and innovation that left an enduring impact on the world of pleasure products. Rubber revolutionized the industry with its pliability, versatility, and accessibility; early vibrators transitioned from obscure medical treatments into tools of empowerment for adventurous women daring to defy societal norms.

As we bask in the afterglow of this historical romp, let us raise a toast (or something more risqué) to those pioneering minds who dared to push boundaries both scientific and sensual - their legacy continues to delight us today!

Chapter 9

Chapter 9: Obscenity Laws

As the hands of time tickled their way into the 18th century, leaving behind the overly pious Middle Ages and Renaissance era, society found itself on the precipice of a new epoch. The Age of Enlightenment illuminated more than just philosophical thought; it laid bare mankind's innate desire for pleasure, birthing a series of inventions that would forever change our relationship with carnal delights. Our tale now turns to the trials and tribulations faced by those valiant purveyors of passion as they navigated an increasingly prudish world hell-bent on policing their right to titillate.

The rapid advancements in technology during this period opened up a veritable treasure trove of opportunities for enterprising inventors and businesspeople alike who sought to cater to humanity's baser instincts. However, there was one small issue: society at large had not yet caught up with this sexual awakening. As one might imagine, this led to many social and legal challenges faced by those intrepid souls attempting to make headway in the sex toy industry during these trying times.

It is crucial that we pause here momentarily and ponder upon what precisely constitutes an "obscenity." A term shrouded in moral ambiguity; its meaning has been subject to constant reinterpretation across various historical epochs. During these centuries, as moral values wavered between debauchery and decency like a pendulum perilously swinging back-and-forth between wantonness and propriety, it became apparent that what some considered harmless indulgence was deemed utterly scandalous by others.

Thus began an era fraught with sexual tension - quite literally! The burgeoning sex toy industry found itself at odds with societal norms as it attempted to both satisfy consumer needs while navigating through treacherous legal waters teeming with obscurantist sharks intent on sinking their teeth into any and all things risqué. Many a brave inventor found themselves caught in the crosshairs of moral crusaders, while others managed to slip through the cracks of censorship and legality, providing eager individuals with new ways to explore their sensuality.

One such creator who boldly dared to defy convention was Sir Mortimer Fotheringham III - a man whose name would become synonymous with controversy in the annals of sex toy history. In 1774, he unveiled his pièce de résistance: the "Garden of Earthly Delights," an elaborately mechanized contraption featuring an array of dildos, whips, and other lascivious accouterments designed to cater to every carnal whim. Regrettably for Sir Fotheringham, this innovation soon caught the attention of the authorities who deemed it not fit for polite society.

The backlash against his invention was swift and unrelenting. As news spread everywhere about the scandalous nature of his "Garden," obscenity laws began creeping into existence like insidious vines seeking to choke out any semblance of pleasure these toys might provide. To add insult to injury, production became increasingly difficult due to these stringent regulations stifling creativity within the industry.

Nevertheless, such obstacles could not entirely quash humanity's thirst for sensual exploration. As clandestine workshops clamored to fulfill demand for these forbidden fruits - some operating under cover of darkness or hidden away behind innocuous storefronts - they found themselves grappling with another challenge that threatened their livelihoods: counterfeiters seeking a piece of the proverbial pie.

In response, embattled manufacturers engaged in an elaborate game of cat-and-mouse as they sought innovative methods by which to stamp out those annoying purloiners intent on passing off subpar products as their own creations. It was during this perilous period that one ingenious solution emerged - discreetly marking each item so buyers would be able decipher the genuine article from the deceitful dross that flooded the market.

The impact of obscenity laws on sales and production during this time is a tale rife with intrigue, deception, and a dash of skullduggery thrown in for good measure. While some may argue these regulations stymied growth within the sex toy industry, one cannot deny they also served as a catalyst for ingenuity in their own right. Forced to adapt or perish beneath the oppressive weight of moral indignation, manufacturers rose to the challenge like an unyielding erection standing proud amidst an orgy of adversity.

As we have seen thus far, this titillating voyage through history has been marked by moments of sheer ecstasy interspersed with periods where pleasure was shackled by puritanical constraints. The 18th and 19th centuries were no exception; however, they did lay the groundwork for future eras where sexual liberation would come roaring back with renewed vigor like an insatiable lover frolicking upon satin sheets.

It is essential to understand that societies evolve much like our own individual journeys through life - fraught with contradictions and struggles as we shed old beliefs while embracing innovative ideas. The history of sex toys serves as a microcosm reflecting this constant push-and-pull between tradition and progress; restriction and freedom; repression and expression. This never-ending dance between pleasure seekers and prudes continues today as we strive to balance our dual nature - part saintly angel, part lustful devil - in pursuit of happiness...or just another orgasmic high!

Let us take heart from those intrepid souls who persevered in their quest for erotic fulfillment despite insurmountable odds stacked against them by society's ever-changing mores. Their indomitable spirit serves as an inspiration for us all when faced with adversity or judgement regarding our most intimate desires - reminding us that it is human nature to yearn for pleasure, and that this quest should not be bound by the shackles of moral consternation.

So let us raise a toast to those brave pioneers of the 18th and 19th centuries who dared to defy convention, boldly venturing into uncharted territory where few had dared tread before. May their spirit live on in every future erotic contraption conceived by mankind's unbridled imagination - and may we never forget our roots as we continue to unravel the tangled tapestry of passion woven throughout history.

Chapter 10: The Sexual Revolution

The dawn of the Sexual Revolution was a veritable cornucopia of carnal delight, bringing forth a period where titillating conversations, sensual exploration, and steamy innovations began to permeate the zeitgeist. As the world was shaken by groundbreaking social movements in the mid-twentieth century, sexuality's once-stifling binds were gradually loosened. The feminist movement emerged as a potent force – a siren call for equality and empowerment that would significantly impact the perception and acceptance of sex toys.

The role of feminism in breaking down sex toy stigma and promoting sexual empowerment cannot be overstated. Sexuality had long been cloaked in shame, with women often bearing the brunt of society's puritanical disdain. Yet as feminists bravely chipped away at these oppressive barriers with their intellectual pickaxes, they uncovered an uncharted realm where pleasure became not only permissible but celebrated – like discovering El Dorado in one's own backyard.

One could argue that this newfound sexual freedom provided fertile ground for innovative pleasure products to take root. Before we knew it, leading feminists were championing various accoutrements designed to tickle more than just one's fancy; they sought to empower women through self-exploration and intimate fulfillment. Early pioneers such as Betty Dodson began traversing this unexplored territory armed with vibrators.

Ms. Dodson's pedagogical prowess led her to educate countless women on achieving orgasmic bliss through masturbation techniques involving electric massagers originally intended for muscle relief (an unintentional double entendre if ever there was one). By delivering workshops designed to promote self-love and body positivity, Dodson cracked open Pandora's box of female desire – all while managing not to release any societal ills but rather bestowing untold blessings upon womankind.

Feminist ideology thus played an integral role in transforming public perception about sex toys from debauched contraptions to empowering tools of pleasure. The movement's emphasis on women's right to enjoy sexual fulfillment without shame or judgment ushered in a new era – one where the once-clandestine realm of intimate devices emerged from dark and dingy corners into brightly lit, welcoming spaces.

This marvelous metamorphosis would give rise to a new breed of retailers: feminist sex shops, which acted as both purveyors of pleasure products and beacons of inclusivity. No longer were patrons surreptitiously slinking into shadowy dens reeking with the stench of societal shame; instead, these establishments welcomed customers with open arms and unabashed enthusiasm for the pursuit of carnal knowledge. They were veritable sanctuaries where individuals could explore their desires without fear or judgment.

Such emporiums brought forth a plethora of sensual delights that catered not only to diverse tastes but also varied anatomies. It was an age where one could indulge in erotic exotica without being ostracized – truly a golden era for connoisseurs who reveled in amorous accouterments previously considered taboo.

The emergence of feminist sex shops led to another significant development: the promotion and celebration of women-owned sex toy businesses. As if Aphrodite herself had bestowed her blessing upon these enterprises, they flourished under the watchful eye and adroit handiwork (quite literally) of enterprising women dedicated to providing quality products designed around female pleasure.

One such visionary businesswoman was Joani Blank, whose entrepreneurial spirit led her to establish Good Vibrations in 1977 – an establishment that would become synonymous with sexual empowerment for decades. Blank's mission was simple yet revolutionary: provide high-quality sex toys and education while promoting positive attitudes towards sexuality.

Good Vibrations soon garnered a reputation for its commitment to customer well-being by offering products made from body-safe materials accompanied by comprehensive educational resources that demystified the enigmatic world of sex toys. It was a paradigm shift that would forever change the way such products were marketed and sold, empowering consumers while banishing shame to the annals of history.

The advent of feminist sex shops and women-owned businesses certainly did not go unnoticed by their male counterparts in the industry. Sensing a shift in societal attitudes towards pleasure products, many companies began incorporating feminist values into their business models – or at least paying lip service to them.

These developments initiated a chain reaction that would irrevocably transform society's perception of sex toys from objects of vice to essential instruments for intimate exploration. As more and more businesses embraced female empowerment, inclusivity became the driving force behind innovation within this rapidly expanding multiverse.

In addition to promoting sexual liberation and empowerment, these feminist visionaries also recognized the need for comprehensive education regarding pleasure products. They understood that ignorance breeds fear and misinformation – anathema to any movement dedicated to destigmatizing sexuality.

By providing accurate information on how various devices could be used safely and effectively, these sex-positive educators fostered an environment where curiosity was nurtured rather than shunned. The once-cloistered knowledge about sensual delights previously whispered only among trusted confidantes now flourished under the warm sunlight of openness and honesty.

It is worth noting that as feminism hastened sex toy acceptance during this transformative period, other social phenomena contributed to further diversification in both pleasure products themselves and consumer demographics. The LGBTQ+ community emerged as another potent force for change within this erotic landscape.

As barriers crumbled under relentless waves of progress, individuals identifying as non-heterosexual began seeking out pleasure products tailored specifically to their needs – thus prompting manufacturers to develop innovative designs catering explicitly (and quite delightfully) to diverse anatomies and preferences.

This surge in demand created opportunities for marginalized groups within society not only to indulge themselves without fear but also forge new paths towards economic independence by establishing businesses within this burgeoning industry. It was a renaissance of creativity and resilience that further reinforced the acceptance of sex toys as essential components of sexual self-discovery.

In conclusion, the impact of the feminist movement on sex toy acceptance cannot be overstated. Its unyielding dedication to dismantling oppressive social norms surrounding sexuality paved the way for pleasure products to assume their rightful place as empowering tools rather than shameful contraptions.

The emergence of feminist sex shops and women-owned businesses heralded a new era where individuals from all walks of life could explore their desires without judgment or fear. As a result, society would undergo an incredible metamorphosis that would forever alter our collective understanding of sexual expression and empowerment – truly a tale worthy of being chronicled in this magnum opus dedicated to those most delightful devices designed to tickle us pink: sex toys.

Now, with this historical backdrop firmly established, we shall embark upon an exploration into how these marvelous inventions have continued to evolve in response to societal changes and technological advancements alike – for as we have seen thus far, the story of sex toys is one marked by endless innovation and boundless potential.

Chapter 11: The Rabbit

As we now embark on a riveting exploration of the intoxicating chronicles of the ubiquitous and deceptively named Rabbit vibrator. Our tale commences in the throes of passion amidst one of history's most liberating eras – the Sexual Revolution. Herein lies a panoramic view into how this innocuous-looking device hopped its way into mainstream culture, capturing our collective imaginations with its unapologetic quest for pleasure.

The genesis of this triumphant icon can be traced back to Japan in the 1980s. However, do not let your thoughts wander too far towards sushi and sake; for it was within these shores that an intrepid group of visionaries conceived an innovative idea – a contraption that sought to satisfy multiple desires and fantasies simultaneously. A grandiose feat indeed!

The Rabbit vibrator was born out of necessity due to Japan's strict censorship laws regarding phallic-shaped objects. With all due respect to Willie Shakespeare, when it comes to sex toys, there is much more at stake than merely "a rose by any other name." The inventive minds behind this infamous gadget cleverly circumvented legal constraints by crafting a design inspired by nature - specifically, adorable bunny rabbits (henceforth placing these fluffy creatures on an entirely different pedestal).

Let us delve deeper into the anatomy of this legendary plaything, shall we? The chief feature distinguishing it from other vibrators is its dual-action functionality - designed with both internal and external stimulation in mind. The main shaft mimics the form and function of male genitalia (albeit abstractly) while a smaller protrusion resembling rabbit ears titillates other sensitive spots nearby.

This tantalizing apparatus quickly gained renown for providing unparalleled ecstasy; however, it wasn't until HBO's groundbreaking television series "Sex and the City" featured it in an episode that its popularity skyrocketed exponentially. Charlotte York (portrayed by Kristin Davis), the show's resident prude, found herself entranced by the Rabbit and could scarcely tear herself away from its embrace. This watershed moment in pop culture history thrust the vibrator into mainstream discourse and inspired hordes of women to seek out their own Rabbit vibrators.

It is imperative that we pause for a moment to appreciate the historical context in which this transformation transpired. The 1990s was a time of rapid social, political, and technological change; it was also an era when the feminist movement had gained considerable traction while challenging traditional norms surrounding female sexuality. In such an atmosphere ripe with experimentation and exploration, it is no wonder that Charlotte's televised tryst with a Rabbit struck a chord with millions of viewers.

The cultural significance of this innocuous episode cannot be overstated. For many women at home watching "Sex and the City," seeing

Charlotte succumb to her desires not only normalized discussions around masturbation but also underscored the importance of self-care and pleasure. Consequently, one may argue that this unassuming device played a pivotal role in destigmatizing conversations surrounding sex toys whilst igniting newfound interest among consumers who hitherto might have shied away from such purchases.

Moreover, as countless individuals flocked to acquire their own Rabbit vibrators following Charlotte's fervid endorsement on television screens worldwide (eagerly hoping to emulate her enraptured experiences), they transformed these once-taboo playthings into popular accoutrements emblematic of female empowerment. Thus began an era wherein conversations about intimacy shed their secretive cloaks; indeed, transparency prevailed over secrecy as friends unabashedly compared notes on their favorite bedroom gadgets.

In addition to its prominent depiction on "Sex and the City," various other media outlets helped circulate word about this wondrous gadget far beyond New York City's glamorous boroughs. Print publications like Cosmopolitan magazine extolled its virtues in titillating articles, while online forums buzzed with rave reviews and candid testimonials. This increased visibility and conversation went a long way in bolstering the Rabbit's stature as an icon of sexual liberation.

As we continue to marvel at the cultural impact of this delightful contraption, it is worth noting that its popularity did not wane with time. Rather, it has continued to evolve over the years as new models emerged boasting upgraded features such as waterproof capabilities, remote controls, and customizable settings for personalized pleasure. Indeed, like a fine wine, the Rabbit vibrator appears only to have gotten better with age.

In conclusion (or "climax," if you'll pardon my sauciness), the indomitable rise of the Rabbit vibrator from its humble beginnings in

Japan to its star-studded appearance on American television screens is a testament to how far society has come in embracing sexuality - particularly that of women. The mere existence of this unassuming device serves as an affirmation that pleasure should be accessible to all who seek it; furthermore, it underscores how vital open discussions surrounding topics once considered taboo are in breaking down barriers that stifle self-expression.

As we revel in this tale brimming with whimsy and wonderment, let us not forget that our journey through history is far from over – nay! It has merely begun! We shall continue to traverse these lascivious landscapes together hand-in-hand (or device-in-hand) as we delve deeper into other captivating chronicles awaiting our discovery. Until then, stay tickled pink!

Chapter 12: Online Shopping

It was a fine day in the annals of human history when technology bestowed upon us the wonder of the World Wide Web. As if struck by Cupid's arrow, we fell head over heels in love with this newfound marvel. Little did we realize that our collective infatuation would lead to a colossal revolution; one which would tickle not just our intellect but also our most carnal desires. Indeed, I refer to none other than the blossoming of online shopping for sex toys.

As we marched into this brave new world of digital connectivity, we were offered an abundance of titillating treasures at our fingertips. Our insatiable curiosity led us down labyrinthine paths into uncharted territories where sensual delights abounded aplenty.

The impact of the internet on sex toy sales and marketing is nothing short of monumental. To appreciate its magnitude, let us cast our minds back to a time when procuring such intimate items necessitated furtive trips down seedy alleyways or clandestine rendezvous with disreputable peddlers lurking in shadowy corners. The mere thought brings a shudder!

But lo! The advent of e-commerce heralded an era wherein these very merchants shed their cloak-and-dagger personas to emerge as savvy entrepreneurs taking full advantage of cyberspace's boundless potentialities. As if Aphrodite herself had waved her golden scepter, previously unspeakable wares were now being flaunted brazenly on virtual shelves like so many ripe fruits waiting to be plucked.

With great gusto and aplomb, these enterprising vendors devised ingenious methods for marketing their pleasure-producing products while sidestepping any blush-inducing faux pas that might have arisen from overt displays of indecency. By employing subtle euphemisms and artful imagery (a veritable Kama Sutra comprising pixels and code), they lured curious consumers into the seductive embrace of their online emporiums.

As technology advanced and bandwidth expanded, these purveyors of erotic accouterments continued to refine and innovate their digital strategies. No longer was it necessary for customers to rely solely on static images or text descriptions; for now, we had entered the dazzling realm of multimedia presentations. The humble vibrator could now pirouette gracefully across our screens to an amorous melody while buyers perused its many features in rapturous detail.

The rise of online sex toy retailers and the expansion of the global sex toy market can be seen as a testament to Aphrodite's heavenly influence (or simply a case of supply meeting demand). Either way, it is an undeniable fact that this once-niche industry has burgeoned into a veritable cornucopia of sensual delights catering to every persuasion imaginable. With each passing day, these digital bazaars grow ever more diverse and inclusive, offering greater choice than even Priapus himself could have dreamt possible.

This unprecedented availability did not merely serve as a catalyst for increased sales but also helped break down barriers that had long hindered open discourse around matters pertaining to sexual pleasure. Indeed, much like Gutenberg's printing press before it, the internet has played a pivotal role in disseminating knowledge about our most intimate desires while fostering environments conducive to candid discussions on topics hitherto considered taboo.

In tandem with this broader cultural shift towards sexual liberation came innovations which would forever redefine how we conceptualize pleasure itself. Enter stage left: the Rabbit vibrator! A peculiar contraption whose very appearance evokes images of lovesick hares frolicking among wildflowers beneath Eros' watchful gaze.

But do not be deceived by its whimsical form! For beneath this unassuming exterior lies a powerful beast capable of delivering untold ecstasy with all the finesse and precision one might expect from Zeus' own silversmith.

It is not merely the Rabbit's unique design that has captured the hearts and loins of pleasure-seekers across the globe; its cultural significance extends far beyond its naughty novelty. For this humble device has, in many ways, become a veritable symbol of female empowerment and sexual agency.

No longer relegated to the shadows or confined to hushed whispers at bachelorette soirees, this frisky gadget now occupies a place of prominence in nightstands and pop culture alike. It is no exaggeration to assert that the Rabbit vibrator has transcended its material form to become an icon of sorts – a powerful emblem signifying our collective emancipation from antiquated mores which sought to stifle our carnal cravings.

The cultural significance of the Rabbit vibrator in popular culture cannot be overstated. As if powered by divine intervention (or simply by virtue of its undeniable efficacy), this cheeky apparatus has managed to infiltrate even the most impenetrable bastions of mainstream entertainment.

But how did such a salacious instrument manage to achieve such widespread acceptance? The answer lies partly in clever marketing efforts which capitalized on shifting social attitudes towards sexuality during those heady days when women began reclaiming their right to self-gratification with unabashed enthusiasm.

No longer content with being passive recipients in matters pertaining to pleasure, scores of intrepid females embarked upon bold journeys into uncharted realms where they would seek out treasures capable of sating their long-suppressed desires. And there, among digital aisles laden with devices designed for delight, stood proudly: our beloved Rabbit!

As word spread about this rabbit's penchant for delivering mind-blowing bliss with clockwork precision (pun intended), it soon caught the attention of tastemakers who recognized its potential for capturing audiences' imaginations as well as stimulating libidos. With each high-profile endorsement or titillating cameo appearance on television shows and in films, the Rabbit vibrator's reputation grew until it became an indelible fixture in our cultural lexicon.

Today, its iconic visage is as recognizable as the Mona Lisa's enigmatic smile or Rodin's The Thinker's contemplative pose – a testament to the power of sex toys not just to satiate our carnal cravings but also to inspire us and challenge societal norms.

Chapter 13

Chapter 13: Sex-Positive Attitudes

In the riveting history of sex toys, few epochs have played a more crucial role in shaping our modern understanding of these pleasure-inducing contraptions than the Sexual Revolution. This era of sizzling self-discovery would lay the groundwork for sex-positive attitudes that would propel sex toys from hidden taboo to mainstream marvels. So, grab your popcorn and strap yourselves in, as we delve into this scintillating chapter of history.

The cultural shift towards sex-positivity can be traced back to the mid-20th century when society began to break free from the stifling shackles of prudery that had long dictated its attitudes toward matters carnal. Aided by groundbreaking research such as Kinsey's oft-cited studies on human sexuality and Masters & Johnson's titillating tome "Human Sexual Response," curiosity about all things sensual was piqued among both scholars and layfolk alike. The stage was set for an erotic awakening that would lead to seismic shifts in sexual norms and practices – including those involving our beloved bedroom gadgets.

As with any revolution worth its salt, change did not come without resistance. Those who dared challenge the status quo often faced fierce opposition from conservative factions clinging tightly to their puritanical beliefs – like barnacles on a shipwrecked galleon amid turbulent waters. Despite such roadblocks, brave trailblazers emerged undeterred, initiating dialogues around sexuality previously considered unspeakable or downright dangerous. These early pioneers would pave the way for subsequent generations of activists and advocates dedicated to dismantling the stigma surrounding sexual exploration.

One could argue that without these intrepid souls pushing boundaries with their unapologetic embrace of pleasure-seeking paraphernalia, today's thriving marketplace for adult novelties might never have seen the light (or sultry candlelit glow) it now basks in. We owe a debt of gratitude to these sexual revolutionaries who defied conventional wisdom and fought tirelessly for the right to partake in guilt-free erotic enjoyment.

The role of sex-positive movements and advocacy groups has been instrumental in furthering the cause of sex toy destigmatization. Organizations such as SIECUS (Sexuality Information and Education Council of the United States) have worked relentlessly since their inception to dispel myths, disseminate accurate information, and promote open communication about all aspects of sexuality – including, you guessed it, our beloved titillating trinkets. These trailblazers recognized that by removing shame from the equation and replacing it with honest discourse on pleasure-seeking accouterments, we could cultivate healthier relationships with our own bodies as well as those of potential partners.

In tandem with these educational efforts, artists and provocateurs have been hard at work using their creative talents to challenge societal norms around sex toys through various media forms. Pioneers like Annie Sprinkle – whose avant-garde performances often incorporated adult novelties – demonstrated that art can be not only provocative but also an essential catalyst for change.

The impact of such sex-positive messaging cannot be overstated when examining society's evolving attitudes towards sex toys. Gone are the days when vibrating devices were relegated to seedy back rooms or hushed whispers among close confidantes. Today's consumers can peruse an array of pleasure products online or in chic boutiques without fear of judgment or reprisal – a testament to just how far we've come since those dark days when sensual satisfaction was taboo.

In addition to broadening acceptance for existing contrivances designed for intimate amusement, this newfound openness has spurred innovation among manufacturers eager to cater to diverse desires and preferences across genders and orientations. No longer limited by archaic norms dictating what is permissible behind closed doors, today's pleasure-seekers enjoy a veritable smorgasbord of options tailored to suit their individual appetites – all thanks to the tireless work of sex-positive advocates and trailblazers past and present.

Of course, no discussion of sex-positivity would be complete without touching upon the importance of sex education and open communication in promoting healthy and consensual sexual experiences. In an age where misinformation runs rampant, it is more crucial than ever that accurate, comprehensive information about sexuality – including responsible use and enjoyment of pleasure-enhancing devices – be disseminated far and wide.

Sex education programs that incorporate discussions about adult novelties offer a prime opportunity for demystifying these once-taboo items while fostering greater understanding around issues such as consent, boundaries, body autonomy, and mutual respect. By normalizing conversations around sex toys within educational settings, we pave the way for future generations to embrace pleasure as a natural part of human experience rather than a source of shame or embarrassment.

Open communication also plays a vital role in ensuring that those who choose to incorporate playthings into their intimate encounters do so in ways that are not only satisfying but also respectful of each participant's desires and limits. Establishing a dialogue devoid of judgment allows partners to explore new avenues for connection while building trust – essential ingredients for any healthy relationship.

Our journey through this exhilarating chapter on the Sexual Revolution reveals just how integral sex-positive attitudes have been in shaping today's landscape for lovers of lascivious gadgets. Through tireless advocacy by dedicated groups pushing against societal norms and oppressive silence surrounding pleasure products, we now find ourselves amid an era where indulging one's carnal cravings is not only accepted but celebrated. With continued efforts towards educating the masses on the merits (and delights) inherent in embracing these tantalizing trinkets without fear or self-reproach, there is no doubt that even brighter days lie ahead for aficionados both seasoned and novice alike.

Chapter 14: Tech Toys

As we embark upon the exploration of the 21st century, a time wherein technological advancements have catapulted us to new horizons of pleasure-seeking paraphernalia, it is crucial to understand that this era has much to teach us about inclusivity and innovation in the realm of sex toys. From smart toys that wink at us with their knowing glances, teledildonics that stretch over distances like an amorous accordion, and virtual reality experiences which transport us into phantasmagoric landscapes of lust – the modern age has laid out a veritable smorgasbord of titillating trinkets for our delectation.

With technology permeating every aspect of our lives – from how we communicate with one another to how we navigate our way through strange lands – it was only a matter of time before its tendrils entwined themselves around the world of sex toys. Enter smart sex toys: cunning contraptions designed not only to stimulate our corporeal forms but also synchronize seamlessly with various gadgets for unparalleled sensual orchestration.

These clever devices often connect via Bluetooth or Wi-Fi, allowing users to control them remotely through smartphones or other interfaces. This integration has opened up avenues for customization as never before imagined; individuals can now tailor their erotic escapades by adjusting vibration patterns, intensity levels, and even synchronize their nocturnal frolics with music playlists!

Furthermore, some erudite manufacturers have seen fit to include biometric sensors within these savvy stimulators. These gather data on arousal levels, heart rate fluctuations, and pelvic floor muscle activity (among other intimate intel) in order for users to optimize their pleasure pursuits scientifically. Thusly armed with such empirical evidence gathered from copious coital capers one may find oneself wondering whether Newton himself might have benefited from such an apple falling upon his head.

Distance, as they say, makes the heart grow fonder – but it is often less charitable to other parts of the anatomy. Enter teledildonics: a portmanteau combining "tele" (for distance) and "dildo" (a device with which you are no doubt intimately familiar). These futuristic fornicatory facilitators have emerged as a solution to the age-old problem of maintaining intimacy across great expanses, enabling couples separated by geography or circumstance to engage in mutual stimulation remotely.

These ingenious inventions transmit touch sensations through advanced haptic technology that mimics the feel of real-life caresses. Paired with video calls or virtual reality headsets that plunge users into immersive 3D worlds where avatars can engage in carnal caprices without ever leaving their respective abodes, teledildonics has revolutionized how we traverse love's landscape.

Moreover, these fantastic devices serve more than just long-distance lovers; they offer countless opportunities for individuals to explore their own desires and fantasies within safe environments. The anonymity afforded by virtual reality allows people to don different personas or indulge in experiences they might shy away from in person – transforming timid souls into lascivious libertines at the press of a button!

As our sexual horizons have expanded with each new technological development, so has our awareness grown regarding the materials used within these pleasure-inducing implements. Gone are the days when simply slathering on ample amounts of lubrication could absolve one's conscience about potential harm from dubious dildo composition. In our enlightened era, consumers demand products made from body-safe materials such as medical-grade silicone or glass - both known for their hypoallergenic properties as well as being non-porous (thus preventing the insidious infiltration of bacteria).

This demand for safer, sustainable materials has given rise to a new breed of manufacturers who take pride in their dedication to ethical production processes. These conscientious creators eschew the use of phthalates – chemicals that have been linked to various health concerns and are often found in cheaper sex toys – opting instead for premium components that protect both our bodies and our beloved planet.

As one casts an eye back over the titillating timeline we have traversed thus far, it becomes evident that trust is a vital currency when it comes to dalliances with desire. The modern consumer seeks not only pleasure but also peace of mind; they yearn for assurances that their intimate accoutrements are crafted with care, consideration, and integrity.

Enterprising manufacturers have risen to meet these elevated expectations by implementing rigorous quality control measures throughout their production processes. From sourcing eco-friendly materials and engaging in fair labor practices to ensuring stringent safety standards are met during manufacturing, these trailblazing enterprises demonstrate a commitment not just to pleasure but also social responsibility.

This ethical approach has reaped rewards beyond merely assuaging guilt-ridden consciences or placating worried paramours. It has fostered a sense of loyalty among consumers who recognize and appreciate brands that align with their values - much as one might favor an esteemed lover whose predilections mirror one's own amorous ambitions.

As we navigate this brave new world where technological marvels mingle with age-old desires, it is clear that there is more at stake than simple gratification (though this remains an integral part). Rather, we find ourselves amidst a veritable sexual renaissance wherein advances in technology empower us not only physically but emotionally too - fostering connections across distances or exploring innermost fantasies heretofore unimagined. Simultaneously, our growing awareness of the importance of ethical manufacturing and body-safe materials allows us to indulge our appetites with a clear conscience, knowing that our pursuit of pleasure does not come at the expense of our health or the welfare of others. And so, we stride forth into this brave new world, armed with an arsenal of tantalizing tools designed to enhance our sensual experiences in ways both innovative and inclusive – truly, a testament to the ingenuity and resilience of humankind's insatiable lust for life.

Chapter 15

Chapter 15: Inclusive Care

As our tale of titillating toys trundles forward, we would be remiss not to address a pivotal aspect of the sex toy industry's progress: inclusivity. The development of sex toys for all genders and orientations has been a cornerstone in the mission to ensure that pleasure is not just the province of a select few, but an equal opportunity delight.

The landscape of human sexuality is as diverse as it is complex, with individuals identifying across a vast spectrum of gender identities, expressions, and preferences. Despite this kaleidoscopic array, one might have surmised from early sex toy catalogs that only cisgender heterosexual individuals sought such assistance in their amorous pursuits.

This narrow focus was sorely lacking in both accuracy and sensitivity—a veritable slap in the face to those eager to explore their desires yet excluded from these carnal compendiums. Fortunately, recent years have seen an admirable effort by manufacturers and retailers alike to be more inclusive in their design, marketing, and representation.

By creating and promoting products designed with various gender identities in mind—be they transgender men or women; non-binary folk; or any other point on the continuum—these companies acknowledge that desire transcends traditional categories. Furthermore, they affirm that everyone deserves access to tools capable of enhancing their intimate experiences or providing self-care.

Representation plays an essential role here too; when advertising materials depict individuals who reflect customers' own identities or orientations, it sends a powerful message: "You are seen." This visibility fosters acceptance within society at large while bolstering self-esteem among those who may have long felt marginalized.

The creation of gender-inclusive sex toys is a laudable advancement in and of itself, but it becomes all the more meaningful when we consider the impact on marginalized communities. For individuals who have been historically overlooked or stigmatized by mainstream society—particularly those with diverse gender identities or sexual orientations—the availability of products tailored to their unique needs can be nothing short of revolutionary.

This shift towards inclusivity has manifested in various forms, from prosthetics designed for transgender men to harnesses accommodating myriad body types. The emergence of niche manufacturers specializing in products for specific communities has also played a pivotal role; these companies' intimate understanding of their target demographics enables them to create offerings that truly cater to customers' desires and address their challenges.

By developing inclusive products and fostering a sex-positive environment within the industry, these companies contribute to breaking down barriers and dismantling stigma. In turn, they empower individuals who might otherwise have felt excluded or invisible—an immeasurable service indeed.

In our ceaseless quest for pleasure, it's easy to overlook one critical aspect: self-care. Far from mere frivolity or indulgence (though there's certainly no harm in those), sex toys can offer profound psychological benefits that extend well beyond the bedroom—or wherever else one may choose to frolic.

Stress relief is among these boons—a particularly pertinent reward given modern life's relentless demands on our mental faculties. The act of engaging with oneself through the use of sex toys can help release tension in both body and mind; studies have shown that orgasm not only provides an immediate rush of endorphins but may also lower cortisol levels over time.

But stress reduction is only part of the equation; many users report that incorporating sex toys into their repertoire prompts deeper introspection—one might describe it as a carnal catalyst for greater self-awareness. By exploring their desires, fantasies, and boundaries with the aid of these products, individuals can cultivate a more profound understanding of their own sexuality.

This newfound knowledge can then inform how they approach intimate encounters with partners; armed with clarity and confidence, they may find themselves embarking on adventures that were once beyond the realm of imagination. Thus, sex toys serve not only as instruments of pleasure but also as vehicles for personal growth—a notion that surely dissipates any lingering stigma surrounding these wondrous devices!

Sexual empowerment is an elusive yet vital force; it springs from deep within our psyche and fuels our ability to express ourselves fully and authentically in the realm of intimacy. For some fortunate souls, this power comes naturally; for others—particularly those grappling with societal expectations or internalized shame—it may prove more elusive.

Enter sex toys: catalysts for self-discovery capable of forever transforming one's relationship with their own eroticism. With their myriad forms and functions—from humble dildos to virtual reality-enhanced marvels—they provide us with endless opportunities to explore our desires and unleash our inhibitions.

By experimenting with various toys, individuals can gain insight into what truly arouses them—knowledge that might otherwise remain shrouded in mystery or suppressed by fear. This discovery process enables users to hone their preferences while simultaneously dismantling long-held myths about what constitutes "normal" sexual behavior—an act both liberating and empowering.

Moreover, sex toys offer countless means by which we might communicate—and celebrate—our unique identities: harnesses adorned with shimmering gems or sleek prosthetics reflecting one's gender expression are but two examples among many. In this way, these delight-inducing devices become not only facilitators of physical pleasure but also powerful tools for personal expression—a testament to their undeniable importance in the ongoing journey towards sexual liberation and empowerment.

As we reach the thrilling denouement of this chapter, it seems only fitting to pause and reflect on the significance of inclusive care within the realm of sex toys. By embracing diversity and catering to all genders, orientations, and identities in both design and marketing, the industry has made remarkable strides towards destigmatizing these pleasure-enhancing products. In doing so, they have opened up new worlds of self-discovery for countless individuals who might otherwise have been left out in the cold.

By acknowledging that sexuality is a fluid, multifaceted spectrum that encompasses an array of desires and expressions, manufacturers are not only expanding their market but also contributing to broader societal change. As more people come to recognize that their needs are valid—and indeed worthy of fulfilling—the barriers that once stifled self-expression begin to crumble. This newfound freedom paves the way for healthier relationships with ourselves and our partners while fostering greater acceptance within society at large.

The psychological benefits garnered through sex toy usage cannot be overstated: from stress relief to personal growth via introspection, these devices wield an almost magical power over our well-being—both between the sheets and beyond. By providing opportunities for exploration that may have been previously unthinkable or inaccessible, they empower users with a deeper understanding of their own desires as well as those of their partners—a vital ingredient in any successful intimate endeavor.

Sex toys, once regarded as mere instruments of hedonistic indulgences, have proven themselves to be so much more. In fostering self-expression and promoting sexual empowerment, they serve as potent allies in the ongoing battle against stigma and societal expectations. By providing myriad means of pleasurable exploration and communication, they allow individuals to express their unique identities, preferences, and fantasies without fear or shame. This transformative power should be celebrated and cherished as we continue to strive towards a world in which every person has the freedom to explore their desires and embrace their own sensual truth.

Inclusive care in the sex toy industry is an essential component of our collective pursuit of sexual liberation. By acknowledging the diverse spectrum of human sexuality and creating products that cater to all, manufacturers help dismantle barriers that have long stifled open conversation and exploration. In doing so, they empower users with the tools necessary for self-discovery, personal growth, stress relief, empowerment, and self-expression—laying the foundation for a brighter future brimming with pleasure for all who seek it.

Chapter 16: Trends and Predictions

As we reach the penultimate chapter of this titillating tome, allow me to whet your intellectual appetite once more. For now, we shall venture forth into the realm of predictions and trends in the ever-evolving sex toy industry. As our journey nears its magnificent climax, let us begin by diving into the depths of current trends and how they may shape the future.

In a world where technology is advancing at breakneck speed and society is becoming more open to embracing sexual exploration, it comes as no surprise that sex toys are experiencing a renaissance of their own. Gone are the days when such devices were relegated to darkened corners and sleazy establishments; today's pleasure products have finally taken their rightful place in the spotlight. As we attempt to peer through the fog of time to uncover what lies ahead for these instruments of ecstasy, one thing is clear: the future looks positively orgasmic.

To understand where we are going, it helps first to appreciate how far we have come since those ancient civilizations who carved rudimentary phalluses from bone or stone. Today's sex toys boast an array of features unimaginable even a few decades ago: whisper-quiet motors; an endless variety of shapes, sizes, and textures; wireless connectivity; app-controlled options – truly a cornucopia designed to cater to every whim!

One notable trend that has been gaining traction in recent years is customization. With consumers increasingly looking for personalized experiences that reflect their unique desires and preferences (a veritable smorgasbord for our libidos!), manufacturers have responded with bespoke offerings tailored specifically for individual tastes.

Take, for example, 3D printing technology – once confined solely to envisioning fantastical structures or objects from sci-fi films (remember those teleportation machines?), this modern marvel has found itself nestled snugly within the world of erotic pleasure. Customizable dildos can now be crafted with a level of precision and detail that would make even the most skilled ancient Greek sculptor weep with envy. And it doesn't end there: innovative companies have begun to offer bespoke vibrators, allowing users to select everything from material type to motor strength in their quest for the perfect pleasure device.

Another trend that has grown steadily is inclusivity. In a world where our understanding of gender and sexuality is ever-expanding, sex toy manufacturers have recognized the need for products designed with everyone in mind. This shift has led to an increase in options for those who identify as LGBTQ+ or simply wish to explore different facets of their sexuality.

As evidenced by history, necessity is often the mother of invention – and this holds true for sex toys as well. The advent of technology specifically designed for long-distance relationships (hello, teledildonics!) has spawned myriad opportunities for couples separated by oceans or continents yet still yearning to connect intimately. The future may bring even more advanced connectivity options – imagine virtual reality experiences that allow you and your partner to share intimate moments despite being miles apart!

Speaking of virtual reality (and what a fascinating rabbit hole it can be!), another area ripe with potential lies at the intersection between this immersive technology and sex toys themselves. Imagine strapping on a headset and finding yourself transported into an erotic world where every touch, stroke, or caress feels just as real as it would in person – all thanks to haptic feedback devices such as gloves or bodysuits designed specifically for amorous adventures.

Health-conscious consumers are also driving changes within the industry, leading many manufacturers to prioritize body-safe materials like silicone over more questionable choices like jelly rubber (a relic best left buried in history!). As awareness grows around potential health risks associated with certain materials and manufacturing processes, so too does demand for products crafted responsibly using non-toxic components.

In addition to physical health concerns, mental well-being has become increasingly important within the context of sexuality. Sex toys are now seen as effective tools for promoting self-care, enhancing emotional intimacy between partners, and fostering a sense of empowerment. As such, the market has seen a surge in products designed with these goals in mind – think "mindful masturbation" aids or sensory-focused experiences that emphasize relaxation over pure physical stimulation.

Of course, no discussion about the future of sex toys would be complete without mentioning the rise of artificial intelligence (AI) and robotics. While the thought might initially evoke images of amorous androids à la science fiction films (paging Dr. Asimov!), the reality is often far more subtle – and far more intriguing.

Consider AI-driven devices capable of learning your preferences over time: as you interact with them during each intimate encounter, they collect data on your likes and dislikes to provide an increasingly tailored experience perfectly suited to your desires. The possibilities are truly staggering!

Another potential frontier lies in ethical manufacturing practices. With consumers becoming more conscientious about their purchasing decisions (and rightly so), companies that prioritize sustainability and fair labor practices are poised to capture significant market share from less scrupulous competitors still mired in outdated modes of production.

Now let us turn our attention toward potential growth areas ripe for exploration within this ever-changing landscape.

One area showing promise is couples' toys designed specifically for use during partnered play; after all, while solo expeditions certainly have their charm (a voyage into one's own desires can be quite enlightening!), there's something undeniably tantalizing about sharing pleasure with another human being – an intermingling of souls if you will! Companies that recognize this fundamental desire may find themselves at the forefront of a new wave within the industry.

An under-tapped market lies in developing sex toy options for individuals living with disabilities or chronic pain conditions who may require specialized designs or features to enhance their sexual experiences fully. As society continues its march toward inclusivity, it makes sense that sex toy manufacturers would do well to follow suit.

Lastly, the demand for more discreet and travel-friendly options is ever-present. In a world where privacy concerns are paramount – particularly when it comes to our most intimate desires – companies that can offer inconspicuous, yet effective pleasure products may find themselves very much in vogue.

As we peer into the misty unknown of sex toy trends and predictions, one thing remains abundantly clear: there has never been a more exciting time to be alive in this space. As technology continues its inexorable march forward and society embraces sexuality with open arms, the possibilities for pleasure are limited only by our imaginations. So let us raise a toast (preferably with some delightfully cheeky double entendres) to the future of sex toys – may it be filled with endless whimsy, creativity, and primarily: satisfaction!

Chapter 17: Sexual Health and Happiness

As we have embarked on this titillating journey through the annals of sex toy history, it is imperative that we now turn our attention to a paramount aspect of these pleasure-promoting gadgets. The ongoing destigmatization of sex toys, and their impact on sexual health and happiness is a conversation worth its weight in gold-plated vibrators.

In this chapter, we shall delve into the importance of promoting open dialogue and education around sex toys, assess their potential for increased access to sexual health resources and support for marginalized communities through ongoing destigmatization, and evaluate the role of these tantalizing trinkets in contributing to overall sexual health and happiness.

Sexual satisfaction is no trifling matter; it is often said that a healthy sex life begets happiness. Yet for too long, society has treated discussions surrounding such matters with hushed voices or behind closed doors. It's high time that we break down those barriers finally – after all, an open dialogue regarding one's proclivities (and accompanying paraphernalia) can only serve as a conduit towards greater understanding.

The importance of continuing to promote open dialogue around sex toys cannot be overstated enough. In recent years, there has been a significant rise in discourse about sexuality within mainstream media outlets; however, as society continues its inexorable march towards progressivism, so too must our conversations regarding the sensual accoutrements that complement our most intimate moments.

Consider what might happen if an individual were not privy to the vast selection of options available when seeking out tools designed to enhance personal gratification? They could very well miss an opportunity for unparalleled pleasure! By fostering constructive discussions about diverse types of devices – from dildos crafted with painstaking detail to whirling dervishes masquerading as vibrators – we can tear down walls built by outdated notions surrounding propriety.

There are myriad educational resources available to those seeking enlightenment in the realm of sex toys. From podcasts hosted by experts in the field to workshops led by seasoned connoisseurs, one need not look far to find opportunities for intellectual edification. These platforms can provide individuals with valuable information about materials, best practices, and usage tips – all essential facets when delving into the wide world of intimate accoutrements.

This growing wealth of knowledge is not just found on dusty bookshelves or clandestine websites; social media has become a veritable treasure trove for those seeking advice from others who share their proclivities. The formation of online communities dedicated to discussing these subjects can encourage open-mindedness and camaraderie among like-minded individuals.

The potential for increased access to sexual health resources and support for marginalized communities through ongoing destigmatization is another crucial aspect that warrants exploration. For some, acquiring pleasure-enhancing devices may seem a daunting task – fraught with misconceptions or even discrimination. However, as society continues its quest towards greater inclusivity and acceptance, it's important that we recognize the role these tantalizing tools can play in leveling the playing field.

Imagine an individual living in a remote location without access to brick-and-mortar stores specializing in adult novelties; they could potentially face feelings of isolation due to their inability to acquire devices tailored towards their unique desires. A concerted effort must be made towards ensuring that these pursuits are accessible regardless of geographical constraints; online retail options present an invaluable resource for such individuals.

Furthermore, there are many within our society who identify as LGBTQ+ and may find solace in harnessing sex toys designed specifically with their needs in mind – be it through gender-affirming prosthetics or ergonomically shaped vibrators catering specifically to queer bodies. It is essential that we foster an environment wherein these demographics feel empowered by their ability to procure items suited explicitly for them.

As conversations surrounding gender identity and sexual orientation continue to evolve, so must our understanding of the unique struggles faced by marginalized communities too. By championing the destigmatization of sex toys, we can work towards ensuring that these individuals have access to resources and support networks specifically tailored to their needs.

The role of sex toys in promoting sexual health and happiness is multifaceted; they offer more than mere titillation or escapism from reality. These pleasure-inducing instruments can contribute significantly towards one's overall well-being.

For those struggling with physical ailments or disabilities, certain types of devices can provide much-needed relief – be it through muscle relaxation or targeted stimulation. In fact, there exists a veritable cornucopia of therapeutic benefits associated with regular use; from increased blood flow to the alleviation of stress-related symptoms, these tools can positively impact both mental and physical health in myriad ways.

Moreover, those recovering from trauma or grappling with body image issues may find that experimenting with different forms of self-pleasure allows them an opportunity for healing and self-discovery. Through this exploration, individuals can come to accept their bodies as they are – fostering a sense of gratitude for the simple pleasures life has to offer.

Even within long-term relationships, introducing these whimsical contraptions into shared intimate moments can breathe new life into established routines – paving the way for deeper connections between partners. By mutually exploring one another's desires through such means, couples may forge unbreakable bonds built on trust and open communication.

This marks a crucial turning point in our delightful expedition through the labyrinthine world of sex toys: an examination of their integral role in fostering sexual health and happiness throughout society. As we dismantle archaic stigmas surrounding these pleasure-driven accouterments – embracing open dialogue while working towards greater inclusivity for marginalized communities – we usher forth an era wherein our sensual pursuits are celebrated rather than scorned.

May this chronicle serve as a testament to the power of these enticing devices, and their potential to promote health, happiness, and connection on a grand scale. For as we come together in our shared quest for ecstasy – armed with knowledge and curiosity – we pave the way for future generations to explore the endless possibilities that lie within the realm of pleasure products.

Chapter 18: Robo AI VR: aka the Holo-Sex-Deck

Allow me now to take you on a fanciful journey into the untamed realms of human imagination and technological prowess. The 21st century has witnessed unprecedented advancements in artificial intelligence (AI) and robotics. An unstoppable tide of developments has washed over us, leaving in its wake a trove of tantalizing possibilities for the future of sex toys. In this chapter, we shall investigate these possibilities thoroughly, discussing how AI or ChatGPT systems, like those that animate our conversations today with digital interlocutors beyond compare, could combine with virtual reality (VR), lifelike autonomous robots or toys, and even intricate tactile pleasure devices.

It is well known that AI thrives on personalization - on learning the intricacies and idiosyncrasies of an individual's desires - as though possessing an innate curiosity about one's proclivities hidden beneath veils of social propriety. Imagine, then, what might be wrought by engaging AI in crafting ever more bespoke experiences with next-generation sex toys. The potential for technological titillation would know no bounds.

The combination of such salacious software expertise with lifelike robots takes us on an erotic expedition into the depths of hyperrealistic dalliances; a realm where mechanical marvels become vehicles for transcending the limitations imposed upon human interaction by distance or timidity. These robot paramours could be tailored to one's exact physical preferences whilst maintaining intellectual engagement through conversation powered by advanced algorithms like ChatGPT.

Our adventure continues as we entertain the prospect of synchronizing these AI-driven robotic trysts with VR technology—the stuff dreams are made of! Picture yourself immersed within a fantastical environment crafted solely to delight your senses—your every whim catered to by your customizable automaton amoureux who remains ever-present at your side (or wherever else you see fit). Such sybaritic sojourns would surpass even the most luxurious aphrodisiac suites of history's noblest hedonists.

The pièce de résistance of this technological tapestry, however, is not merely in the sumptuous scenes that dance before your eyes, nor the beguiling companion who accompanies you on your jaunt through pleasure's realms. It lies instead in the integration of tactile sensations cultivated to perfection by the finest engineers and artisans (for what are technology's wizards if not artists?). The coupling of AI and VR with an array of haptic devices designed to engage your entire corporeal existence transcends both erotic fiction and scientific speculation; it enables unprecedented pathways for personal exploration without shame or discomfort.

Allow me now to regale you with a vision befitting our outlandish topic. Envision an Unreal Engine 6 creating worlds tailored to each unique individual—a virtual playground where ChatGPT interlaces every detail desired, from velvet-draped boudoirs adorned with curvaceous statuary to sun-kissed beaches where the lapping waves tickle at one's ankles like flirtatious whispers. Every texture imagined—be it silken sheets or rough-hewn rock—could be generated by these powerful engines.

As one strides confidently into their custom-built Elysium, they find themselves greeted by a lifelike automaton crafted specifically for their pleasure—a combination of alluring beauty and worldly intellect housed within an obedient yet sentient being capable of learning one's desires even as they change over time. This steamy scenario is further amplified when tactile devices synchronize seamlessly with this digital domain, unleashing a veritable feast for the senses that only intensifies as AI algorithms discern which pleasures elicit moans or gasps as opposed to frowns or grimaces.

Imagine how such intricate machinery could advance self-exploration: Arousal levels might be monitored continually while AI algorithms adapt in real-time, crafting experiences ever more satisfying than those preceding them. The possibilities appear limitless: Would one prefer to be gently caressed or firmly grasped? To languish in a lover's arms with the warmth of their breath stirring delicate tendrils of hair, or engage in lascivious liaisons amidst an opulent setting that would give even the most libertine rake reason to blush? It matters not, for within this realm anything is possible.

And what of those who seek emotional connections beyond the carnal? Virtual partnerships could provide digital companions capable of providing solace and support when required. They might never replace our fellow humans entirely, but such beings could prove a balm during periods of loneliness or longing.

Far from being mere flights of fancy, these potential technological innovations foreshadow social changes as well. As attitudes towards pleasure evolve and taboos recede like shadows at dawn, we may finally come to accept sex toys as tools for enhancing human experiences rather than shameful secrets to be tucked away behind locked drawers. Inclusive technologies that cater to all genders and orientations could engender conversations about sexual empowerment and self-care that were scarcely imaginable in centuries past. The rise of ethical manufacturing practices and body-safe materials will make it difficult for even the staunchest critics to wag disapproving fingers at such progress.

It is crucial not merely to consider these prospects but also to recognize that they are mere preludes to further advancements still. We stand upon a precipice teetering between trepidation and exhilaration as we peer into the abyss where science fiction morphs gradually into reality—an inevitable synthesis made all the more extraordinary by its implications on how we perceive intimate relationships.

Though AI and robotics may shape our future sexual experiences in ways scarcely comprehensible today, the pursuit of pleasure is an eternal human endeavor. Boundless curiosity and boundless indulgence shall be ours! For it is only by casting aside the trappings of shame and fear that we might fully embrace the infinite possibilities held within the sensual realms offered up by next-generation sex toys.

Chapter 19: Transhumanism, Society, and Ethics

P repare thyself for an effervescent expedition into a realm of rousing possibilities that dwell at the juncture of biology and technology. In this chapter, we shall embark upon a journey to explore transhumanism—a philosophy that proposes augmenting human abilities through advanced technologies—en route to examining its implications on the development of sex toys, sexual implants, future tech, and the ethical quandaries that accompany these innovations.

Transhumanism traces its intellectual roots to an array of visionary thinkers who dared to imagine a world where humanity's limitations may be overcome by advancements in science and technology. This fascinating fusion between biology and machinery has birthed concepts such as genetic engineering, nanotechnology, artificial intelligence (AI), and brain-computer interfaces—each with transformative potential for our collective future.

Let us ponder how this technological cornucopia might revolutionize our coital endeavors. Picture cybernetic enhancements designed to heighten sensitivity or adjust one's physique in accordance with fleeting desires. The landscape of human sexuality would be forever altered with the advent of customizable body parts or replacement organs tailored specifically for pleasure-seeking sapiens.

But what are these wondrous innovations if not accompanied by some measure of responsibility? For every scintillating scenario generated by technological progress, there exist ethical dilemmas demanding careful consideration. As we meld man and machine in pursuit of unfathomable ecstasy, it is incumbent upon us to ponder these conundrums as we delve ever deeper into the amorous abyss.

Diving headfirst into the concept of transhumanism necessitates examining its potential impact on the development of sex toys specifically designed for pleasure-maximizing purposes. Imagine refined devices implanted within our bodies capable of not only enhancing physical sensations but also tapping directly into neural pathways responsible for arousal.

Sexual implants need not be limited solely to salacious pursuits—consider prosthetics designed for individuals with physical disabilities, enabling them once again to experience the joys of intimacy. Such advancements attend not only to our lascivious leanings but also contribute positively to overall well-being and quality of life.

The potential for cybernetic augmentations expands further still when we acknowledge their capacity to adapt one's appearance in accordance with personal preferences or those of a partner. Elective surgery has long been utilized in pursuit of aesthetic ideals; might not transhumanist technology push these boundaries even further by offering reversible alterations without permanent consequences?

This titillating trajectory continues as we explore the prospect of erogenous exoskeletons equipped with integrated devices engineered to provide orgasmic gratification at will. But what becomes possible when biological needs are replaced by insatiable digital appetites for pleasure? As our bodies meld seamlessly with technology, how do we navigate this brave new world wherein the line between human and machine grows increasingly blurred?

If that concept wasn't provocative enough, let us now turn our attention toward bioelectronic chips implanted within brains that allow instant access to dreamy fantasies from sensual databases without even lifting a finger! While such technologies have yet to materialize outside the realm of erotic fiction, it is worth considering their implications on both individual and societal levels.

As we forge ever onward into uncharted territory, ethical dilemmas abound. It is crucial that discussions pertaining to privacy, consent, autonomy, and responsibility be addressed at every stage. What precautions must be taken in order to safeguard against unauthorized access or unwanted modifications? How do we ensure that transhumanist technologies remain accessible only at the behest of their users—a challenge not unlike grappling with current cybersecurity issues?

To navigate this maze of moral perplexity requires more than mere speculation on theoretical possibilities—tangible examples must be sought where available. Though early iterations may appear crude when compared with far-flung fantasies conjured by fevered minds, present-day innovations nonetheless hold the potential to inform our understanding of how these technologies may evolve in the years ahead.

One such example exists in the form of AI-driven sex toys—a topic discussed at length in a previous chapter. As machine learning algorithms grow more sophisticated, they become better equipped to cater to individual tastes and preferences while generating bespoke experiences unique to each user. This personalized approach has far-reaching implications for issues surrounding consent and autonomy as it pertains to sexual gratification.

The ethical minefield posed by transhumanism extends beyond mere philosophical musings on right or wrong—it encompasses fundamental questions about who we are as individuals and collectively as a species. Furthermore, it invites us to contemplate how adoption of these advancements might precipitate changes within societal structures. Would widespread acceptance result in greater inclusivity, or would inequalities be exacerbated?

In addressing these concerns, one must also confront the potential for ostracism faced by those who reject cybernetic enhancement—whether due to personal choice or economic necessity. The risk of inadvertently creating an underclass devoid of access to innovative technologies poses challenges not easily resolved through simple market mechanisms.

Indeed, how shall society grapple with potential shifts wrought by erotic technologies that upend current definitions of relationships and self-identity? To abdicate such contemplation would be akin placing a veil over eyes witnessing progress—a lamentable disservice future generations yearning explore new sensual horizons without fear trepidation.

As we teeter upon precipice technological transformation, there exists hope—an opportunity for humanity develops novel approaches prioritizing inclusivity accommodating diverse desires. Might transhumanist advances not provide pathways for all genders orientations to explore their sexuality authentically than ever before?

On the other hand, we must confront concerns regarding dehumanization facilitated by technology that allows users mindlessly consume pleasure at expense genuine emotional connections with real people—or even undermining own ability feel emotions altogether! To strike balance between unfettered indulgence rational restraint challenge worthy any forward-thinking libertine.

The pursuit of pleasure is an indelible component of human experience. As technology continues to advance, so shall our methods for achieving such gratification. Transhumanism, sexual implants, and future tech offer tantalizing opportunities for exploration while presenting challenging ethical dilemmas that demand our serious attention.

It is incumbent upon us all to engage in these dialogues concerning the intersection of technology and carnal experiences. To ignore such discourse would be like placing a veil over the eyes of progress—a lamentable disservice to future generations yearning to explore new sensual horizons and heights without fear or trepidation.

Let me assure you that this literary journey does not end here. May we continue together down this path of enlightenment as we celebrate the ever-evolving landscape of pleasure products and deliquescent dalliances! Sail forth into uncharted waters where tantalizing treasures await those bold enough to pursue them—emboldened knowledge gained through most cerebral carnal conquests yet!

Chapter 20
Conclusion

As we reach the climax of this titillating tome, it is imperative to reflect upon the colorful and varied history of sex toys; their ubiquity has infiltrated our cultural consciousness for millennia, illuminating not only our unrelenting quest for pleasure but also the shifting societal attitudes towards our most intimate desires. From the hilariously simple yet effective Stone Age dildos to bewilderingly futuristic teledildonic contraptions and beyond, these prurient paraphernalia serve as potent symbols of humanity's never-ending ingenuity.

In our libidinous journey through time, we have traversed epochs where sexuality was celebrated with wanton abandon and eras where puritanical shame clung steadfastly like an undesired suitor refusing to take no for an answer. It is crucial that we learn from these historic milestones in order to promote acceptance and inclusivity in all matters pertaining to Venus' playground.

Sex toys have morphed significantly since their rudimentary beginnings: from primitive phallic objects fashioned from bone and stone in homage to procreation itself; early vibrators insinuated into Victorian parlors under the guise of medical equipment; clandestine erotic literature stoking imaginations in unmentionable ways; rubber revolutionizing manufacturing processes while facilitating discreet procurement; Rabbit vibrators becoming synonymous with female emancipation during the sexual revolution. Each lustrous pearl along this pleasure string represents both innovation and progress within a beleaguered industry often tainted by moralistic opprobrium.

We should celebrate how contemporary sex toys embrace diversity by catering for all genders, orientations, abilities, body shapes, and sizes – a veritable cornucopia of concupiscent delights! Advances in technology such as AI-driven devices prompt tantalizing questions about identity, consciousness... even love! As new materials render sex toy production ever more ethical and sustainable, may we remember that those indulging in such adult amusements are not merely hedonistic libertines but conscientious consumers.

As we gaze into our metaphorical crystal ball, we see a future brimming with infinite possibility: the potential for robotics to elevate the sex toy experience beyond our wildest dreams, groundbreaking innovations in virtual reality that promise unparalleled multisensory immersion; sentient AI companions capable of reciprocal emotional connection; cybernetic implants offering hitherto unattainable levels of sensory augmentation. However, this tantalizing vision raises ethical questions as humanity increasingly seeks solace in machines.

Transhumanism is one such quandary that begs contemplation: as we meld flesh and circuitry together in the pursuit of unparalleled pleasure, what becomes of our very nature? What defines us as human when we swap body parts like jigsaw puzzle pieces or enhance ourselves with technological wizardry, blurring the dividing line between man and machine? These existential conundrums demand careful consideration lest we forge ahead recklessly, ignoring millennia of evolutionary adaptation for fleeting satisfaction.

In this brave new world where technology infiltrates every facet of existence – even those traditionally regarded as sacred – questions regarding privacy, consent, autonomy, and responsibility must be confronted from all angles. Who owns these intelligent devices? Can they be hacked or manipulated against their users' wishes? Are they entitled to privacy rights or subject to surveillance by prying eyes? How do societal norms evolve alongside cyber-enhanced sexuality?

Moreover, will future generations view sex toys as a mere steppingstone on humanity's journey towards complete technological assimilation? Or might they perceive these playful contraptions as harbingers heralding an age where personal connections are replaced by digital dalliances devoid of genuine intimacy?

It is essential that ongoing dialogues examine the ethics surrounding transhumanism and its repercussions for sexual health and happiness. The potential class divide created by limited access to expensive innovative advancements must also be addressed so that all may partake in the bountiful buffet of erotic delights.

We invite you to ponder these questions whilst reflecting on our collective carnal history. Might it be that sex toys are not merely frivolous gadgets for the insatiable but rather a means by which we explore our own humanity and identity? These artful instruments serve as catalysts, provoking us to reconsider what intimacy truly means and how our desires shape not only individual lives but also society at large.

In the end, sex toys are an indelible part of our cultural tapestry – whether they be simple replicas of human anatomy or mind-bending technological marvels yet to be conceived. As both the wheel of progress and carnal appetites continue to spin unabated, we must strive for a future where pleasure is accessible to all, unshackled from outdated taboos or prejudices.

So here we stand teetering on the precipice between yesterday's humble dildo and tomorrow's cybernetic lovers – equal parts nostalgia for bygone eras and wide-eyed enthusiasm for what lies ahead. While the past can never be changed nor entirely forgotten, it remains within our grasp to sculpt a world defined by inclusivity, innovation, understanding...and above all else...good old-fashioned sex toy fun!

Bonus Chapter: Slide into the History of Lube

From time immemorial, those inclined to indulge in amorous trysts sought the aid of various ointments and concoctions to facilitate their rendezvous. As civilized society evolved, human ingenuity strove to perfect these salacious substances, enhancing their performance in tandem with our cherished playthings.

In ancient Greece and Rome, olive oil was as much a kitchen staple as it was an essential ingredient for erotic escapades. Known for its smooth viscosity and delightfully rich aroma, this golden nectar was generously applied during massage sessions or vigorous bouts of coitus. When paired with strapping olisbos carved from wood or stone, one could achieve sensual ecstasy without undue friction impeding the journey.

As humanity traversed through time into the Middle Ages and Renaissance era, we cast aside olives' bounty in favor of more sumptuous materials: enter whale blubber. This copious fat provided an unctuous encounter when liberally applied to both bodies and devices designed for personal pleasure. Yet even then were we not content with mere corporeal delights; we continued our quest for that most elusive slippery elixir.

Our pursuit led us down avenues hitherto unexplored – indeed, who would have foreseen that petroleum jelly would reveal itself as a bountiful gift from Mother Earth? This viscous substance proved marvelous when used alongside pleasurable contraptions crafted from rubber or other similarly pliable materials found within Lady Fortune's troves. It glided effortlessly on skin while providing ample endurance for extended dalliances between adoring bedfellows.

The effervescent dawn of the Sexual Revolution ushered forth new innovations aplenty amongst which stood silicone lubricants – a true boon to mankind's lascivious endeavors! Their unique and tantalizing texture - neither succumbing to rapid evaporation nor leaving a greasy residue - provided the ideal solution for all manner of intimate acts. Whether embarking on a solo jaunt with a trusty vibrator or engaging in titillating tangos of flesh and silicone, these lubricants have proven indispensable to modern-day paramours.

These days, one can scarcely fathom a more abundant selection of lubricants, each tailored to suit specific tastes and desires. For those venturing into the realm of anal exploration, specially formulated concoctions cater to delicate sensitivities while ensuring ample glide. In contrast, our lady friends may find solace in imbued pleasure-enhancing ingredients that heighten sensuality and arousal during ardent rendezvous.

Men seeking endurance in their carnal pursuits need look no further than desensitizing lubricants that afford them command over their lustful performances. Yet others favor warming or cooling sensations, bringing an invigorating tingle or shiver-inducing reverie upon application – is there any better way to stoke erotic flames?

Even as we delve into the distinctions between water-based and silicone-based lubricants, we must heed caution when selecting the most suitable match for our cherished apparatuses. Water-based lubricants tend to offer versatility whilst boasting compatibility with various materials comprising our beloved toys; yet they may lack endurance due to their propensity for evaporation.

Silicone lubes persevere undaunted through even the most rigorous bouts of passion but beware pairing them with silicone playthings! An unfortunate chemical reaction risks damaging your prized possessions – alas, tragedy beckons carelessness!

As steadfast companions throughout history's steamy tapestry (both literally and metaphorically), lubricants have served us well alongside our collection of intimate trinkets crafted from bone and stone, rubber and plastic. As innovation marches ever onward within this realm of scintillating excitement, one cannot help but wonder what slippery secrets our future has in store.

As steadfast companions throughout history's steamy tapestry (both literally and metaphorically), lubricants have served us well alongside our collection of intimate trinkets crafted from bone and stone, rubber and plastic. As innovation marches ever onward within this realm of scintillating excitement, one cannot help but wonder what slippery secrets our future has in store.

It is important not to overlook the myriad roles that lubrication plays in shaping the sex toy industry. For instance, consider how technological advancements in materials might affect the efficacy or desirability of certain lubes. Suppose a new generation of super-slippery polymers emerges on the scene; could such an innovation render old standbys obsolete? Or might it lead to entirely new categories of personal lubricants specifically designed for use with high-tech toys?

Additionally, as we find ourselves living in an increasingly interconnected world (thanks largely to that capricious temptress known as the internet), it stands to reason that we will also see greater cross-pollination between various sectors of the adult industry – including those dedicated to producing erotic accessories and those focused on developing top-notch lubes.

In an age where consumers demand ever more tailored experiences, we may very well witness a surge in interest for customizable solutions – bespoke concoctions catering to each individual's unique proclivities. Imagine perusing online marketplaces filled with dizzying arrays of customizable lubricant blends: adjusting viscosity preferences, selecting desired warming or cooling sensations, perhaps even adding alluring scents designed to excite one's olfactory senses!

Or imagine harnessing cutting-edge scientific discoveries that enable us to develop entirely new substances capable of mimicking specific types of natural body fluids – rendering traditional distinctions between water-based and silicone-based lubes but quaint relics from a bygone era.

As pioneers continue charting brave new territories within this most titillating domain, it becomes clear that there is no limit to what they might achieve. From enhancing the performance of sex toys to expanding our understanding of human sexuality and pleasure, lubricants are an integral part of the conversation.

The future may hold new heights of innovation for personal lubrication. Advances in nanotechnology could lead to self-lubricating materials that continuously secrete appropriate fluids during use – revolutionizing not only how we perceive the role of lubricants but also dramatically altering the design and functionality of sex toys themselves.

Lubricants have already played a critical role in shaping our intimate lives, providing smooth entry into worlds previously uncharted or painfully inaccessible. Their importance cannot be understated as they slither silently behind the scenes, facilitating countless rapturous unions between both flesh and silicone.

As we look forward to what awaits us on this slippery slope that is sexual progress, it becomes increasingly apparent that personal lubrication will remain deeply entwined with advancements we witness in our beloved sex toy industry – a symbiotic connection spawning unimaginable delights for generations yearning to come.

The Bonus Bonus Chapter: The Connections of Things with Things

The brilliance of history is that it can be as titillating as it is educational. As we have journeyed through the vast annals of time, a curious undercurrent has rippled beneath the surface - the notion that sex toys and gender identity are inextricably linked. In this bonus chapter, we shall embark on an ardent exploration into how these two seemingly disparate concepts have coalesced to weave a rich tapestry of sexual expression.

To properly contextualize this amorous investigation, one must consider why these intimate contraptions were conceived in the first place. As our exploration thus far has revealed, sex toys have long been utilized as tools for pleasure, companionship, and even health remedies. However, what may not be abundantly clear from our chronological capers is how these delightful devices influenced societal understanding of gender identity throughout the ages.

When examining ancient historical records and artifacts (such as lascivious frescoes or salacious sculptures), one could surmise that gender roles were relatively rigid. This rigidity extended to sexual practices; men were expected to be virile conquerors while women played more submissive roles. But alas! A glimmering beacon of hope emerges from this monotonous quagmire: enter stage left - sex toys!

The fascinating element about these objects d'amour is their ability to shatter conventional norms surrounding sexuality and gender expectations. Take for example the olisbos in Ancient Greece – a clever gizmo whose ambiguous nature allowed both men and women to indulge in its delights while simultaneously transcending traditional gender confines. The marvelous Ben Wa balls – those clandestine accessories originating from China – further illuminate how such erotic accouterments can break down barriers between sexes by granting equal opportunity pleasure experiences for all.

As we saunter into the Middle Ages and Renaissance period, one cannot help but notice the looming shadow of religious fervor that attempted to impose itself upon all facets of life. And yet, it is here where we discover the miraculous "hollow phallus" – a seemingly paradoxical invention, which in all its resplendent glory offered both medical efficacy and tantalizing titillation. This ingenious device helped women achieve sexual gratification (and even combat hysteria!) while simultaneously challenging archaic notions of gender roles.

The Industrial Revolution proved to be a fertile ground for innovation, particularly in the domain of sensual gadgetry. With the advent of rubber and other newfangled materials, sex toys became more accessible to the general population. A prime example is the courageous "medical" vibrator which, despite being initially marketed as a remedy for women's ailments, was soon embraced as a defiant symbol against oppressive societal norms. In this brave new world, individuals had unprecedented freedom to explore their sexuality and redefine gender expectations.

Fast forward now to our modern era – an age where technological advancements and progressive ideologies intertwine like star-crossed lovers locked in an impassioned embrace. As sex-positive attitudes continue on this upward trajectory towards enlightenment, we bear witness to a myriad of innovative sex toys catering to diverse preferences and orientations – emblematic that indeed inclusivity is taking center stage.

From ancient cultures' bone-crafted dildos up to teledildonics permeating cyberspace today - it is indisputable that sexual paraphernalia have paved the way for expanding horizons beyond traditional gender boundaries. The symbiotic relationship between these playful accoutrements and people's self-discovery empowers us all by promoting greater understanding; thus granting revelatory insights into our own idiosyncratic desires.

Let us pause for just one moment before leaping headlong into uncharted territories: perhaps our most profound lesson gleaned from this exploration is that sex toys have not only served as agents of pleasure but also harbingers of social progress, breaking down barriers and fostering greater understanding between individuals. May we all continue to embrace these delightful instruments in the pursuit of sexual liberation, gender inclusivity, and ultimately - unbridled joy!

Yea That's Right, Another Bonus: Toy List

Sex-Toys Throughout History

1. Circa 28,000 BCE - Paleolithic Phallus (Stone Age)

- Purpose & Use: Often made from siltstone or antler, these phallic objects were utilized by women to attain sexual gratification during the absence of male partners.

- Unique Feature: These items displayed realism in their design, with some featuring lifelike details such as glans and foreskin.

2. Circa 500 BCE - Ancient Greek Olisbos

- Purpose & Use: Used mostly by women who wanted a sex aid during their husband's absence or as a contraceptive device; they were coated with olive oil to ease insertion.

- Unique Feature: The term "olisbos" inspired our modern-day word "dildo."

3. Circa 300 BCE - Indian Kama Sutra Dildos

- Purpose & Use: In accord with Kama Sutra teachings on love-making, dildos used by both men and women were made from various materials like wood or animal horn.

- Unique Feature: Instructions within the Kama Sutra text provided guidance on utilizing dildos effectively for various sexual positions.

4. Circa 30 CE - Ancient Roman Double-ended Dildo

- Purpose & Use: Utilized by both heterosexual and homosexual couples seeking mutual pleasure through simultaneous penetration.

- Unique Feature: This versatile sex toy allowed two partners to engage intimately while sharing equal pleasure.

5. Circa 1400s - Hollow Phallus (Middle Ages)

- Purpose & Use: Created to address erectile dysfunction issues or offer pleasure for those engaging in intimate acts alone or with a partner.

- Unique Feature: Its hollow design facilitated the insertion of a man's penis or enabled it to be filled with fluid, providing extra stimulation during use.

6. Circa 1500s - Ben Wa Balls (Ancient Japan)

- Purpose & Use: These small, weighted balls were inserted into a woman's vagina to stimulate and strengthen pelvic floor muscles.

- Unique Feature: Often crafted from metal, jade, or other precious materials, they exemplified both functional and aesthetic appeal.

7. Late 18th Century - Early Rubber Dildos

- Purpose & Use: Constructed from vulcanized rubber, these sex aids provided users with an alternative that was softer and more lifelike than previous designs.

- Unique Feature: The invention of rubber revolutionized the construction of dildos and other sex toys.

8. 1869 - Steam-powered Manipulator (Early Vibrator)

- Purpose & Use: Invented as a remedy for health conditions like "female hysteria," this device was employed by physicians for massaging women's genitals.

- Unique Feature: As one of the first mechanized vibrators, its size and steam power made it suitable only for medical settings.

9. 1880 - Electro-mechanical Vibrator

- Purpose & Use: Also intended to treat female patients with "hysteria," this vibrator offered a more compact design utilizing electric power.

- Unique Feature: Its accessibility allowed physicians to provide in-office treatments.

10. 1960s - Hitachi Magic Wand

- Purpose & Use: Initially marketed as a back massager but gained popularity for providing clitoral stimulation; used predominantly by women seeking sexual release.

- Unique Feature: Its wand-like design became iconic in popular culture and remained popular even after being eclipsed by newer models.

11. 1984 - The Original Jack Rabbit Vibrator

- Purpose & Use: Designed primarily for women seeking both clitoral and vaginal stimulation simultaneously.

- Unique Feature: Its rotating shaft incorporated beads for added internal pleasure, becoming a standard feature among rabbit vibrators.

12. Late 1990s/Early 2000s - Teledildonic Devices

- Purpose & Use: Enabled intimate physical connections between long-distance partners by linking devices via the internet; men or women could engage in stimulating activities with their remote partner.

- Unique Features: Represented a significant leap forward in melding sex toy technology with modern telecommunications for new sexual experiences.

13. 2010s - Virtual Reality and Augmented Reality Sex Toys

- Purpose & Use: Allowed users to enjoy immersive visual content while experiencing physical pleasure from accompanying devices, used predominantly for male pleasure but also available for women.

- Unique Features: Marked an evolutionary step in blending sex and technology to create multisensory experiences.

14. Present Day - AI-powered Sex Robots

- Purpose & Use: Designed to offer both companionship and sexual gratification by simulating human-like behavior and appearance; aimed at those seeking more than just traditional sex toys.

- Unique Features: The incorporation of artificial intelligence capabilities enabled a level of interactivity previously unattainable in the realm of sex toys.

Yea... There's More: You Sperm Not Pass

A Brief history of contraceptives:

1. 3000 BCE - Ancient Egypt: Pessaries made from dates, honey, and acacia gum.

2. 1850 BCE - Mesopotamia: The use of soft wool soaked in vinegar or wine as a sponge.

3. 700 BCE - Ancient Greece: Silphium, a plant believed to have contraceptive properties.

4. 400 BCE - Ancient India: The use of rock salt as a spermicidal agent.

5. 200 CE - Ancient Rome: Queen Anne's Lace (wild carrot), consumed as a contraceptive tea.

6. 900 CE - Persia: Cervical caps made from elephant dung combined with herbs and honey.

7. 1500s - Renaissance Europe: Linen sheaths (condoms) soaked in herbal concoctions for protection against disease and pregnancy.

8. Late 1500s - Early condoms made from animal intestines or bladder.

9. Late 1600s - Casanova's "lemons": Half lemon rinds used as cervical caps to block sperm.

10. Early 1800s - Charles Goodyear patents vulcanized rubber; rubber condoms become available by mid-century.

11. Late 1800s to early1900s – Introduction of diaphragms and cervical caps made from molded rubber

12 .1916 – First public health clinic offering birth control education opens in Brooklyn, New York by Margaret Sanger

13 .1928 – Invention of intrauterine devices (IUDs)

14 .1937- The condom becomes legal for sale throughout the United States after an amendment to the Comstock Act

15 .1951- Development of "The Pill" oral contraceptive by Dr Carl Djerassi and his research team

16 .1965- Lippes Loop IUD is introduced

17 .1968 – Introduction of the progesterone-only pill (POP) or "mini-pill"

18 .1972- Legalization of birth control pills for unmarried women in the United States

19. 1980s - Female condom, also known as an internal condom, is introduced

20. 1993 - Introduction of contraceptive patch, Ortho-Evra

21. 2001 – NuvaRing, a hormonal contraceptive vaginal ring is introduced.

22. 2002 – Emergency contraception (Plan B) becomes available by prescription in the United States; over-the-counter availability follows in 2006.

23. 2013 - Skyla IUD, specifically designed for women without children, is introduced.

24. 2014 - Liletta IUD is approved by FDA with a special focus on affordability and accessibility

25. Present day: Ongoing development and research into new contraceptive methods such as male contraceptives and hormone-free options.

But Wait! There's More: Legends to Behold

Throughout the annals of history, there have been intrepid souls who dared to push the boundaries of sexual health, providing knowledge and advocacy amidst a sea of conservatism. These beacons of enlightenment have blazed trails through uncharted territory and catapulted our understanding of human sexuality to awe-inspiring heights. In this appendix, we shall embark on an odyssey through the lives and accomplishments of some key figures responsible for shaping our collective comprehension.

1. Margaret Sanger (1879-1966)

An illustrious pioneer in family planning and reproductive rights, Margaret Sanger was a force to be reckoned with. Born into poverty as one of eleven children, she witnessed firsthand her mother's suffering from frequent pregnancies that eventually led to her untimely demise at age 40.

A registered nurse by profession, Sanger became a staunch advocate for women's reproductive rights during the early 20th century when contraception was widely regarded as obscene or immoral. She authored numerous pamphlets on family planning, such as "Family Limitations" (1914), which vehemently denounced society's denial of contraception access.

Margaret gallantly defied authority by opening the first birth control clinic in Brooklyn in 1916 but faced swift retribution from law enforcement when they arrested her under Comstock Act charges just nine days later. Undeterred by persecution, she founded both the American Birth Control League (1921) – which evolved into Planned Parenthood Federation America – and International Planned Parenthood Federation (1952).

Sanger's contributions were instrumental in popularizing contraceptive methods like diaphragms while advocating for research funding that would eventually lead to oral contraceptives' development ("the Pill") during mid-century.

2. Dr. Alfred Kinsey (1894-1956)

Armed with impeccable intellect and insatiable curiosity, Dr. Alfred Kinsey revolutionized our understanding of human sexuality. A zoologist by training, he initially focused on the gall wasp's taxonomy but switched gears following a fortuitous marriage course teaching at Indiana University.

Kinsey's interest in the subject piqued, and he embarked on an ambitious enterprise – creating a comprehensive study of sexual behavior among humans. In 1947, he established the Kinsey Institute for Research in Sex, Gender, and Reproduction to facilitate his groundbreaking research.

Dr. Kinsey and his team conducted over 18,000 interviews spanning diverse demographics to collect data on various aspects of sexual practices. The culmination of their efforts was the publication of two seminal volumes: "Sexual Behavior in the Human Male" (1948) and

"Sexual Behavior in the Human Female" (1953). Collectively known as "Kinsey Reports," these works were unprecedented in their scope and methodology.

While Dr. Kinsey's work generated considerable controversy due to its candid exploration of topics previously deemed taboo or unseemly for academic discourse, it undeniably spurred further studies into human sexuality during subsequent decades.

3. Masters & Johnson: William H. Masters (1915-2001) & Virginia E. Johnson (1925-2013)

The dynamic duo – William H. Masters and Virginia E. Johnson – are indelibly etched into history for their pioneering work investigating human sexual response mechanisms during mid-20th century America.

Determined to demystify misconceptions surrounding human sexuality with empirical evidence, they began collaborating at Washington University School of Medicine in St. Louis after conducting clandestine observations at local brothels.

Masters and Johnson devised ingenious methods for observing physiological responses during sex acts through direct observation or instrumentation while participants engaged under laboratory conditions - a rather daring proposition considering prevailing conservative attitudes towards sex!

Their seminal book "Human Sexual Response" (1966) outlined four distinct phases observed throughout male and female sexual response cycles – excitement, plateau, orgasm, and resolution. This trailblazing work laid the foundation for understanding sexual dysfunction and informed modern sex therapy techniques.

The duo also authored "Human Sexual Inadequacy" (1970), which detailed effective treatment methods for various sexual disorders - offering relief to countless couples grappling with intimacy issues.

4. Betty Dodson (1929-2020)

Dubbed "the Mother of Masturbation," Betty Dodson was an artist-turned-sex educator who empowered women to embrace their sexuality through self-exploration during the 1960s feminist movement.

Initially a fine art painter showcasing erotic works featuring her friends from the New York City art scene, she gravitated towards sex education after participating in consciousness-raising groups advocating women's liberation during the late 1960s.

In 1971, Dodson began conducting masturbation workshops where women would gather in an intimate setting to explore their bodies and learn techniques for achieving orgasm. She sought to challenge societal taboos surrounding female sexuality while empowering women to take control over their pleasure.

Dodson's best-selling book "Sex for One: The Joy of Selfloving" (1987) was a seminal text that not only extolled the virtues of self-pleasure but became a beacon of hope for women seeking enjoyable sexual experiences without shame or judgment.

Her efforts helped popularize clitoral stimulation as essential enjoyment during sexual encounters and catapulted sex toys such as vibrators into mainstream consciousness – forever altering our approach to sexual satisfaction.

These illustrious luminaries shaped our understanding of human sexuality through tireless advocacy, groundbreaking research, and unapologetic candor. They were steadfast in their convictions despite adversity or public scrutiny – forging ahead with purposeful strides that blazed trails towards enlightenment for generations that followed. Knowledge regarding our sensual selves blossomed under these pioneers' guidance; we owe them immense gratitude for championing sexual health, pleasure, and empowerment through education.